Essentials of Antimicrobial Pharmacology

A Guide to Fundamentals for Practice

PAUL H. AXELSEN, MD

University of Pennsylvania School of Medicine
Philadelphia, PA

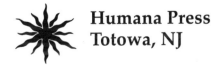

Humana Press
Totowa, NJ

Preface

Antibiotics have cured countless diseases and have saved countless lives. The stellar success of these "wonder drugs" over the past six decades has led to their widespread use (see accompanying table) and this, in turn, has driven the development of many therapeutic options. As our options increase, however, so does the complexity of therapeutic decisions and the risks associated with antibiotic use. The risks to individual patients include life-threatening adverse reactions, treatment failures due to errors in choice of therapy, and treatment failures due to antimicrobial resistance. The risk to institutions and entire populations is the development of organisms that are resistant to all available agents. An understanding of antimicrobial pharmacology is necessary to minimize these risks, and it is for this reason that antimicrobial pharmacology is a critical component of the medical school curriculum.

This guide is derived from the lecture notes prepared for second year medical students at the University of Pennsylvania School of Medicine. These notes have evolved through the efforts of both faculty and students to gage what *can* be assimilated in the midst of an overwhelming amount of other material, and what *must* be assimilated about this subject to understand the general literature of medicine. If we have been successful, then this text contains the information that is essential for medical students to know at the conclusion of their preclinical studies, as well as the information that practicing physicians must know to read the current literature of medicine and remain up-to-date. Pharmacists, nurses, and even business analysts should also find that this is the information they need to understand new developments in the field.

In keeping with its intended role as a "guide" (rather than a textbook for a first-time introduction to the subject), the text is intentionally succinct in style and format. It is a secondary tool that will be most effectively used as a reference, as a review aid, or—as used at Penn—in conjunction with a didactic lecture series. The tables and figures (including figure captions and chemical structures) are provided only to assist in assimilating the text; they should not be regarded as essential to an understanding of the subject.

The author thanks the many expert friends and wise colleagues who offered advice or encouragement in the course of developing lecture notes, and at various stages of text preparation: P.J. Brennan, Helen Davies, Paul Edelstein, Neil Fishman, Ian Frank, Harvey Friedman, Al Goldin, Marilyn Hess, Rob Roy MacGregor, Greg Poland, David Relman, Harvey Rubin, Mindy Shuster, Jeff Weiser, and students in the Pharmacology Graduate Group at the University of Pennsylvania.

As an initial attempt to define an essential body of knowledge about antibiotic pharmacology, the contents of this volume are subject to revision. Suggestions for inclusion or omission are welcome.

Paul H. Axelsen, MD

Note: Most information about currently marketed antibiotics presented in the tables is derived from the National Drug Code Directory updated on March 31, 2001 by the United States Food and Drug Administration. Readers are referred to http://www.fda.gov for more recent updates.

Antibiotics Among the 200 Most Commonly Prescribed Medications in 1999 (From www.rxlist.com)

Rank	Generic Name	Trade Name
9	Amoxicillin	Trimox
16	Azithromycin	Zithromax (Z-Pack)
20	Amoxicillin/Clavulanate	Augmentin
25	Amoxicillin	(generic)
28	Ciprofloxacin	Cipro
29	Cephalexin	(generic, manufacturer #1)
33	Amoxicillin	Amoxil
34	Trimethoprim/Sulfamethoxazole	(generic)
35	Clarithromycin	Biaxin
51	Azithromycin	Zithromax
69	Fluconazole	Diflucan
79	Levofloxacin	Levaquin
82	Cefprozil	Cefzil
98	Penicillin VK	Veetids
102	Cefuroxime	Ceftin
107	Clotrimazole/Betamethasone	Lotrisone
131	Mupirocin	Bactroban
135	Amoxicillin	(generic)
145	Penicillin VK	(generic)
146	Neomycin/Polymyxin/Hydrocortisone	Neomycin/Polymyxin/Hydrocortione
152	Cephalexin	(generic, manufacturer #2)
158	Erythromycin	Ery-Tab
184	Tobramycin/Dexamethasone	Tobradex
188	Terbinafine	Lamisil

Contents

1 Introduction

1.1 Measures of Antibiotic Effect

Antibiotics are natural products that selectively kill or at least inhibit the growth of microorganisms. This narrow definition has been expanded by popular usage to include synthetically or semisynthetically produced antimicrobial agents, as well as antiviral agents and even antiparasitic agents directed against macroscopic organisms.

The pharmacological strategy underlying the therapeutic use of antibiotics involves exploiting biochemical differences between an infecting organism and the host. These differences enable an antibiotic to target the infecting organism and impair one of its critical biochemical processes without harming the host. For any given clinical situation, some antibiotics will be effective and reliable, while others will be ineffective or unreliable. It is misleading to classify antibiotics as being either "strong" or "weak" because the relative effectiveness of different antibiotics varies with the clinical situation. Therefore, the notion of antibiotic "strength" has little meaning. Rather than the strength, or even the potency of an antibiotic, it is more important to consider four other measures of antibiotic effect.

First among these measures is *spectrum of activity*. Antibiotics are classified as being narrow spectrum or broad spectrum depending on the number of different bacterial species against which they exhibit useful activity. A broad-spectrum antibiotic is not necessarily advantageous, because narrow-spectrum agents are often just as effective, and sometimes even more effective at killing bacteria than broad-spectrum agents.

From: *Essentials of Antimicrobial Pharmacology*
By: P. H. Axelsen © Humana Press, Inc., Totowa, NJ

A second important measure of antibiotic effect is *bacterial sensitivity*. Sensitivity is measured by assessing the ability of a bacterial strain to replicate following antibiotic exposure (see Section 1.4). Permanent loss of replicative ability implies that an antibiotic is "bacteriocidal," while temporary loss with the resumption of growth and replication following removal of the antibiotic implies that it is "bacteriostatic." Whether an antibiotic is bacteriocidal or bacteriostatic depends on the organism, antibiotic concentration, duration of exposure, and the circumstances of the infection. Bactericidal activity can be important in some clinical situations, but it is not always, or even frequently necessary for therapeutic efficacy.

A third important measure of antibiotic effect is *therapeutic index*. This is the ratio of the minimum concentration likely to produce an adverse effect to the minimum concentration needed to produce the desired effect. There are many instances in which drugs with a higher therapeutic index are preferable over drugs that are more potent. Many host factors have the potential to alter the therapeutic index.

A fourth measure of antibiotic effect is the *ability to penetrate* and reach the infecting organism. Antibiotics are unique among pharmacological agents in that their site of action may be in any body compartment, or simultaneously in multiple compartments. Delivery of antibiotic to the site of infection is often the most difficult challenge of antibiotic therapy, and treatment failures may often be attributed to a failure of the antibiotic to reach the site of infection. This measure, therefore, must be of paramount concern when planning antibiotic therapy.

1.2 Antibiotic Administration

Oral administration is the most common and often the simplest route by which to treat patients with antibiotics **(Fig. 1.2, top)**. It is also the most direct route when targeting antibiotics to infections within the gastrointestinal tract (e.g., helicobacter, pseudomembranous colitis), but gastrointestinal absorption is a major barrier for many antibiotics targeted against systemic infections. The fractional amount of an oral dose that ultimately reaches the bloodstream is its "bioavailability." Bloodstream infections (septicemia) are rarely treated with orally administered antibiotics because these infections are often

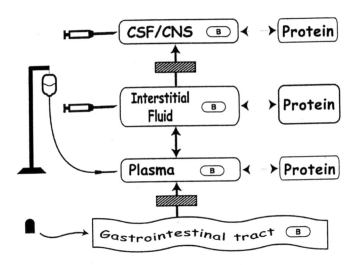

Common routes of systemic antibiotic administration.

There are selective penetration barriers between the GI tract and the plasma, and between the interstitial fluid and the CSF/CNS. In each compartment, active antibiotic is in rapid exchange with inactive protein-bound antibiotic.

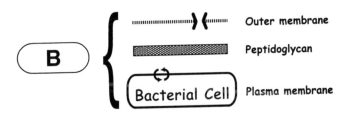

Antibiotics targeted against Gram-negative bacteria must penetrate an outer lipid membrane to reach the cell wall peptidoglycan. This is facilitated by porins - water-filled protein channels. Most antibiotics can readily penetrate the peptioglycan of Gram-negative and Gram-positive bacteria, but they often rely on carriers or transport mechanisms to penetrate the plasma membrane.

Fig. 1.2

life threatening, and the assumed bioavailability of a drug may be reduced for a variety of patient-specific reasons.

Intravenous therapy circumvents bioavailability problems, and is usually preferred for bloodstream infections, or whenever the bioavailability of an orally administered antibiotic is inadequate or in doubt. In most cases, intramuscular injections are just as effective at delivering antibiotic to the bloodstream as intravenous administration. This is because intramuscular injection delivers the antibiotic to the interstitial fluid compartment, and there is little barrier effect between the interstitial compartment of well-perfused tissues and the intravascular space.

Successful delivery of antibiotics to the blood compartment by whatever route is no assurance that adequate amounts of drug will ultimately be delivered to the site of infection because there may be other significant barriers between the blood compartment and the infected compartment. To overcome such barriers, it is sometimes necessary to instill antibiotic directly into an infected compartment, for example, intrathecal administration to bypass the blood–brain barrier.

1.3 Distribution and Elimination

Within the blood, freely dissolved drug and protein-bound drug are in rapid exchange **(Fig. 1.2, top)**. Nonetheless, they behave as if they are in different compartments because protein-bound drugs are unable to either leave the plasma/extracellular space or exert any antimicrobial activity. For this reason, it may be important to distinguish between total and free concentrations when assaying the blood level of an antibiotic.

Some antibiotics are indifferent to the blood–brain barrier and readily pass from the bloodstream into the central nervous system (CNS). In other cases, this barrier is virtually impenetrable. In still other cases, this barrier is impenetrable in the absence of inflammation, but sufficiently penetrable in the presence of inflammation to enable effective treatment.

The biliary and urinary tracts are regulated compartments with stringent physiological control over the entry of antimicrobials into these spaces **(Fig. 1.3)**. Within each of these spaces, however, crystalline or quasicrystalline "stones" may exist into which antibiotic

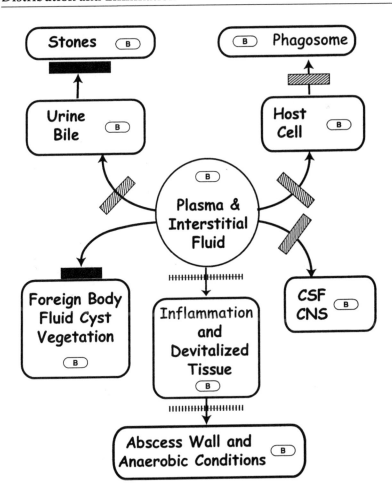

Barriers to antibiotic penetration

From the plasma and interstitial fluid, antibiotics must traverse selective barriers en route to infections in the urine/bile, in the CSF/CNS, and inside host cells. Biliary stones, most foreign bodies, fluid cysts, and vegetations present virtually impenetrable barriers to antibiotic penetration. Antibiotics may be inactivated by inflammation or in anaerobic conditions, or they may be unable to penetrate devitalized tissue or abscess walls.

Fig. 1.3

penetration is virtually nil. Entry into other compartments such as joint spaces and bursae is less stringently regulated, but may nonetheless present significant barriers to penetration. Bone and skin are distinct compartments that concentrate some antibiotics and exclude others.

Prosthetic graft material, fluid cysts, endovascular vegetations, and the glycoproteinaceous "slime" produced by some organisms constitute nonvascularized material that precludes virtually all antibiotic penetration. Cell membranes are impenetrable to many antibiotic classes, and organisms that locate within phagocytic vacuoles are protected by at least two such membranes. Infecting organisms may be situated within an abscess, and abscesses themselves may be situated within a mass of inflamed, poorly perfused, or devitalized tissue. These conditions also prevent the penetration of many antibiotic classes.

Finally, the membranes or cell wall components of the bacterial cell may prevent an antibiotic from penetrating to intracellular sites of action within the microorganism **(Fig. 1.2, bottom)**. In some cases, the cell membranes of microorganisms have pump mechanisms that must be functional for antibiotic penetration, or that actively pump out any antibiotic that gains entry.

Most antibiotics are eliminated from the body into either the urinary or the gastrointestinal tract. It is important to know the mode of elimination so that dosage adjustments may be made if renal or hepatic function is impaired. Prior to elimination, they may be chemically altered. Chemical alteration by the body usually results in an increase in the water solubility of a drug, and this tends to facilitate elimination. Chemical alteration most often destroys the antibiotic activity of the compound, although in some cases activity is significantly increased.

1.4 Sensitivity Testing

There are no antibiotics for which it can be said that the precise "lethal event" is fully understood. Rather, it is more typical that antibiotic action induces a cascade of biochemically dysfunctional processes and a loss of the ability to replicate. The loss of the ability to replicate is the characteristic that is measured when estimating antimicrobial effect, and this point need not coincide with the cessation of metabolic activity in the microorganism.

A distinction is made between the minimum concentration of an antibiotic needed to inhibit growth (the minimum inhibitory concentration or MIC), and the minimum concentration needed to kill an organism (the minimum bactericidal concentration or MBC). However, it usually is not clear how quantitative differences in antibiotic concentration are mechanistically linked to qualitative differences in result (inhibition vs killing). Furthermore, qualitative differences may vanish with long durations of exposure because the ability of many antibiotics to kill microorganisms is a function of both time and concentration. Thus, higher concentrations can reduce the duration of exposure needed to kill a microorganism, and longer exposures can reduce the concentration of a drug needed to kill a microorganism.

The broth dilution approach may be used to determine either an MIC or an MBC (**Fig. 1.4.1**). To determine the MIC of an antibiotic against an organism, the organism is simply inoculated into tubes of culture broth containing various concentrations of antibiotic. The lowest antibiotic concentration that inhibits growth is the MIC. To yield meaningful results, this test must be performed with standard broth formula, incubation conditions, and inoculum size. To determine the MBC of an antibiotic against an organism, the organism is inoculated into tubes of culture broth containing various concentrations of antibiotic as in an MIC determination. After a period of time, samples from each tube are removed and inoculated into antibiotic-free media. The lowest antibiotic concentration that prevents subsequent growth in the antibiotic-free media is the MBC. Owing to their cost as well as difficulties in standardization and interpretation, MBC determinations are not routinely performed on clinical specimens.

Agar diffusion or "disk diffusion" tests are performed by overlaying a thin agar slab with live organisms, and then overlaying a paper disk that contains a known amount of antibiotic (**Fig. 1.4.2**). The antibiotic slowly diffuses out of the disk, eventually distributing evenly throughout the agar. As antibiotic diffuses out of the disk, however, regions in the agar close to the disk experience a relatively high peak concentration of antibiotic. Regions further from the disk experience progressively lower peak concentrations. For regions in the agar in which the integrated antibiotic concentration over time is above a characteristic threshold, the growth of organisms on the agar will be inhibited, and this will be visible as a clear "zone of inhibition"

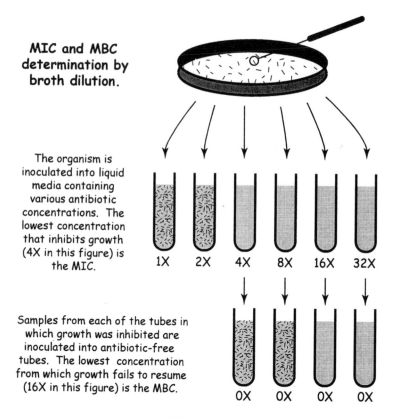

MIC and MBC determination by broth dilution.

The organism is inoculated into liquid media containing various antibiotic concentrations. The lowest concentration that inhibits growth (4X in this figure) is the MIC.

1X   2X   4X   8X   16X   32X

Samples from each of the tubes in which growth was inhibited are inoculated into antibiotic-free tubes. The lowest concentration from which growth fails to resume (16X in this figure) is the MBC.

0X   0X   0X   0X

Fig. 1.4.1

around the disk. The more susceptible an organism is to the antibiotic, the larger the zone of growth inhibition. The zone diameter is translated into a MIC by comparing its size to results obtained by broth dilution methods.

The potential for synergy when using antibiotic combinations may be evaluated either by agar diffusion or by broth dilution methods. One cannot reliably predict synergistic action between any given pair of antibiotics; in all but a few well described situations, it must be assessed using the specific infecting organism. True synergy occurs when the activity of an antibiotic combination exceeds the sum of the

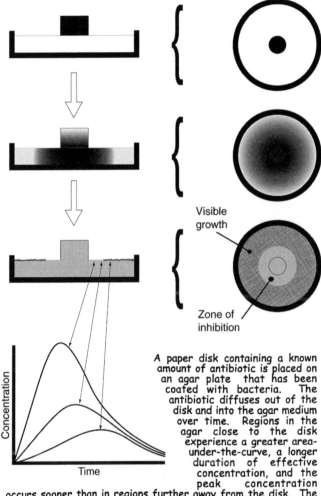

Visible growth

Zone of inhibition

A paper disk containing a known amount of antibiotic is placed on an agar plate that has been coated with bacteria. The antibiotic diffuses out of the disk and into the agar medium over time. Regions in the agar close to the disk experience a greater area-under-the-curve, a longer duration of effective concentration, and the peak concentration occurs sooner than in regions further away from the disk. The diameter of the "zone of inhibition" around the disk in which bacteria do not grow is a complex function of these and other factors, but it is usually possible to correlate this diameter with an MIC obtained by broth dilution methods. The simplicity and low cost of this method makes it advantageous over broth dilution methods for most clinical laboratories.

Fig. 1.4.2

individual activities of each antibiotic. Merely demonstrating that two antibiotics exhibit additive (nonantagonistic) antimicrobial effects does not constitute a demonstration of synergy.

Post-antibiotic effect (PAE) is defined as the period of time that growth remains inhibited after exposure and removal of an antibiotic. This definition implies that the initial exposure was inhibitory but not lethal. Long PAEs are sometimes used to rationalize dosing intervals that allow blood levels of antibiotic to become relatively low between doses.

1.5 Dose–Response Relationships

Sensivity testing is of undeniable utility in predicting the likelihood of success with a given treatment plan in many clinical situations. Nevertheless, the significance of specific numerical results obtained from sensitivity testing is controversial and frequently misunderstood. One reason for this is that blood levels of an antibiotic must be corrected for the fraction that is protein bound and thus inactive. Another reason is that achieving the MIC of an antibiotic in the blood is no assurance that the infecting organisms will be exposed to this concentration in the infected body tissue. Differences in pH and ion content, as well the presence of serum factors and inflammatory cells, may alter bacterial sensitivity to an antibiotic compared to that observed *in vitro*. For these reasons, MIC determinations are more reliable at demonstrating resistance than they are at demonstrating susceptibility.

A third point of confusion about MIC determinations arises because different antibiotics exert their effects by different mechanisms. Antibiotics that bind reversibly to their target sites (e.g., antiribosomal, antifolate, and antitopoisomerase agents) tend to exert greater effects at higher concentrations. Therefore, one achieves the desired result at the MIC, but this result may be more rapidly or more completely achieved at concentrations above the MIC. The overall effect of such an antibiotic dose often correlates best to the integral of the concentration over time. This is frequently referred to as the area-under-the-curve (AUC), where the curve is a graph of the concentration vs time **(Fig. 1.5)**. The calculation of AUC/MIC is frequently used to normalize this information for antibiotics of differing potency.

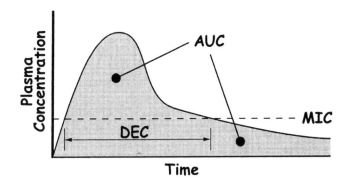

The area under the curve or AUC is the area of the graph of the plasma concentration of an antibiotic vs. time. The duration of effective concentration or DEC is the length of time that the plasma concentration exceeds the MIC. The effectiveness of antibiotics that bind reversibly to their targets correlates best with the AUC of the drug, whereas the effectiveness of antibiotics that bind irreversibly to their targets tends to correlate better with the DEC.

Fig. 1.5

In contrast, antibiotics that bind irreversibly to their targets (e.g., β-lactams) do not tend to exert greater effects at higher concentrations. In these cases, therefore, the effect of an antibiotic dose relates to the duration of time that antibiotic concentrations exceed the MIC: the duration of effective concentration (DEC). In these cases, the effectiveness of the antibiotic is maximal at a concentration near the MIC, and it does not become greater at concentrations higher than the MIC. This notwithstanding, one usually administers much higher doses of an antibiotic to ensure adequate concentrations in all affected body compartments at all times during therapy.

1.6 Resistance

Antimicrobial resistance is especially likely to emerge as a therapeutic problem when widespread usage is combined with suboptimal dosing. This combination of practices is common in two settings. One is the unnecessary treatment of common viral illnesses with broad-spectrum antibiotics, in tandem with poor patient compliance. Another is the addition of antibiotics to animal feeds for growth promotion. Both of these situations apply selective pressure under conditions that permit efficient mutation, rearrangement, and exchange of genetic information. This genetic information is frequently exchanged between species via plasmids, so that the presence of resistance among nonpathogenic organisms represents a reservoir from which pathogenic organisms may acquire resistance.

Physicians must understand and anticipate resistance patterns whenever initiating therapy. These patterns will vary at different institutions and in different communities. Physicians must also assume a role in preventing resistance, by curtailing the inappropriate use of antibiotics and encouraging patient compliance. In the hospital setting, help in doing this is increasingly available in the form of hospital formulary controls that restrict the use of antibiotics in those settings, and expert surveillance systems that track laboratory results and administered therapeutics. To improve patient compliance with especially serious public health problems such as tuberculosis, directly observed therapy (known as DOT) programs are proliferating to monitor and, in some cases, force compliance with prescribed therapy.

2 Antibacterial Agents

2.1 Cell Wall Active Agents (Table 2.1.1)

Bacterial cell walls in both Gram-positive and Gram-negative bacteria contain peptidoglycan. Peptidoglycan precursors are synthesized intracellularly and attached to carrier molecules for export from the cell. Following export from the cell, specific enzymes catalyze transglycosylation reactions in which the peptidoglycan precursors are transferred from their carrier molecules to existing polyglycan chains. Once transferred, other specific enzymes catalyze transpeptidation reactions in which two polypeptide segments are joined. In this manner, a densely crosslinked molecular mesh is created.

The specific chemical composition of peptidoglycan can vary widely between different bacterial species, but it tends to be chemically homogeneous within any one species. Compounds that inhibit individual enzymes involved in peptidoglycan synthesis, or mutations that render individual enzymes inactive give rise to morphologically distorted bacterial cells. This demonstrates the role of peptidoglycan in maintaining bacterial shape. In addition to enzymes that synthesize peptidoglycan, bacteria produce lytic enzymes that remove the crosslinks formed during transpeptidation. Complexes composed of lytic and synthetic enzymes enable bacteria to sever and reform crosslinks in such a way as to permit growth while preserving cell wall integrity **(Fig. 2.1.1)**.

From: *Essentials of Antimicrobial Pharmacology*
By: P. H. Axelsen © Humana Press, Inc., Totowa, NJ

Table 2.1.1

Currently Marketed Bacterial Cell Wall Biosynthesis Inhibitors

Subclass	Generic name	O	IV	IM	T	Trade names
Natural penicillins	Penicillin G	X	X	X	X	Penicillin,[a] Truxcillin, Pfizerpen
	Penicillin G benzathine			X		Bicillin L-A, Bicillin C-R[a] Permapen
	Penicillin G procaine			X		Wycillin, Bicillin C-R[a]
	Penicillin V	X				Pen, Penicillin,[a] V-Cillin, Veetids, Penicillin-Vk, Beepen, Penicillin, Truxcillin-Vk
Aminopenicillins	Ampicillin	X	X	X		Unasyn,[a] Principen, Amficot,[a] Omnipen
	Amoxicillin	X				Amoxil, Amoxycillin, Amficot,[a] Moxilin, Amoxocillin, Amoxicot, Augmentin,[a] Trimox, Sumox
	Bacampicillin	X				Spectrobid
Antistaphylococcal (β-lactamase-resistant) penicillins	Nafcillin		X	X		Nallpen
	Oxacillin	X	X	X		Bactocill
	Dicloxacillin	X	X			Dycill, Dynapen
Broad-spectrum antipseudomonal penicillins	Carbenicillin		X			Geocillin
	Mezlocillin		X	X		Mezlin
	Piperacillin		X	X		Zosyn,[a] Pipracil
	Ticarcillin		X	X		Ticar, Timentin[a]
First-generation cephalosporins	Cefadroxil	X				Duricef
	Cefazolin		X	X		Kefzol, Ancef
	Cephalexin	X				Keftabs, Keftab, Keflex, Biocef
	Cephapirin		X	X		Cefadyl
	Cephradine	X				Velosef

		O	IV	IM	T	
Second-generation cephalosporins	Cefaclor	X				Ceclor
	Cefamandole		X	X		Mandol
	Cefmetazole		X			Zefazone
	Cefonicid		X	X		Monocid
	Cefotetan		X	X		Cefotan
	Cefoxitin		X	X		Mefoxin
	Cefprozil	X				Cefzil
	Cefuroxime		X	X		Kefurox, Zinacef
	Cefuroxime axetil	X			X	Ceftin
	Loracarbef	X				Lorabid
Third-generation cephalosporins	Cefdinir	X				Omnicef
	Cefixime	X				Suprax
	Cefoperazone		X	X		Cefobid
	Cefotaxime		X	X		Claforan
	Cefpodoxime proxetil	X				Vantin
	Ceftazidime		X	X	X	Ceptaz, Tazidime, Tazicef, Fortaz
	Ceftibuten	X				Cedax
	Ceftizoxime		X	X		Cefizox
	Ceftriaxone		X	X		Rocephin
Fourth-generation cephalosporins	Cefepime		X	X		Maxipime
Carbapenams	Imipenem		X	X		Primaxin[a]
	Meropenem		X	X		Merrem
Monobactams	Aztreonam		X	X		Azactam
Glycopeptides	Vancomycin	X	X			Vancoled, Vancocin

[a]Multicomponent product

O, oral; IV, intravenous; IM, intramuscular; T, topical, including preparations applied to skin, eyes, and ears

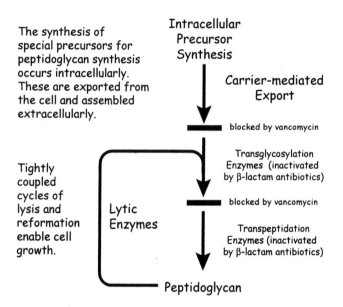

The synthesis of special precursors for peptidoglycan synthesis occurs intracellularly. These are exported from the cell and assembled extracellularly.

Intracellular Precursor Synthesis

Carrier-mediated Export

blocked by vancomycin

Tightly coupled cycles of lysis and reformation enable cell growth.

Lytic Enzymes

Transglycosylation Enzymes (inactivated by β-lactam antibiotics)

blocked by vancomycin

Transpeptidation Enzymes (inactivated by β-lactam antibiotics)

Peptidoglycan

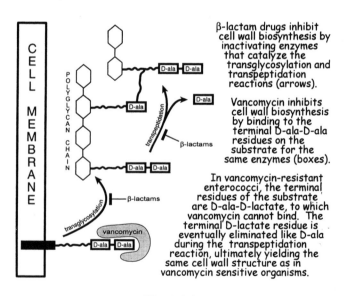

β-lactam drugs inhibit cell wall biosynthesis by inactivating enzymes that catalyze the transglycosylation and transpeptidation reactions (arrows).

Vancomycin inhibits cell wall biosynthesis by binding to the terminal D-ala-D-ala residues on the substrate for the same enzymes (boxes).

In vancomycin-resistant enterococci, the terminal residues of the substrate are D-ala-D-lactate, to which vancomycin cannot bind. The terminal D-lactate residue is eventually eliminated like D-ala during the transpeptidation reaction, ultimately yielding the same cell wall structure as in vancomycin sensitive organisms.

Fig. 2.1.1

Beta Lactams

Identity

All antibiotics in this class possess a β-lactam ring **(Fig. 2.1.2)**. A "lactam" is an amide (a C=O group adjacent to an NH group) within a ring. The prefix β indicates that the ring is comprised of four atoms. Different β-lactam subclasses differ in the kind of ring fused with the β-lactam ring. Different groups attached to these rings distinguish individual drugs within each subclass, altering the pharmacokinetic properties and antimicrobial activity of the parent compound.

Mechanism of Action

β-Lactams are unstable compounds with chemically strained four-atom rings that become more stable when the ring is opened by cleavage of the CO–NH bond. When this occurs, the open ring form typically binds to proteins via its C=O group. This reaction is called "acylation," and it may be compared to the release of tension in a safety pin upon opening. β-Lactam antibiotics specifically and permanently acylate the active site of the enzymes that catalyze the transglycosylation and transpeptidation reactions involved in peptidoglycan synthesis. Collectively, these enzymes are known as penicillin binding proteins, or PBPs. The lethal event is probably the continued activity of lytic enzymes **(Fig. 2.1.1)** that are not inhibited by β-lactam compounds, and the consequent loss of cell wall integrity.

Activity

One might expect that any bacterium with a peptidoglycan cell wall would be susceptible to the action of β-lactam drugs. However, differences among bacteria in the types of enzymes used to synthesize peptidoglycan and a variety of other factors result in wide variations in susceptibility to different drugs **(Table 2.1.2)**.

Administration, Metabolism, and Elimination

The bioavailability of β-lactam antibiotics is highly variable, and adequate blood levels cannot always be attained by oral administration. Due to active secretion by cells lining the proximal renal tubules, in addition to glomerular filtration, natural penicillins have serum half-lives as short as 30 min. Active secretion can be inhibited by concomitant administration of probenecid.

Imipenem (but not meropenem) is degraded by an enzyme in the proximal renal tubule into nephrotoxic products. For this reason,

All β-lactam antibiotics have a β-lactam ring . . .

. . . and acylate the active sites of target enzymes.

Opening of a β-lactam ring is associated with the release of bond-angle strain. The release of this strain may be compared to the release of energy that occurs when a safety pin is opened.

Major subclasses differ in the type of ring adjacent to the β-lactam ring, and different "R" groups distinguish different drugs within a subclass. R groups determine the pharmacokinetics and metabolism of a drug, as well as its spectrum of antimicrobial activity.

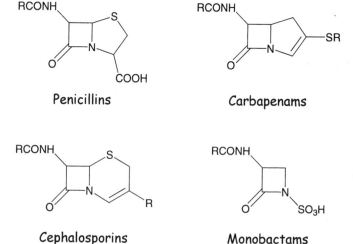

Fig. 2.1.2

it is administered concomitantly with an inhibitor of this enzyme, cilastatin. All β-lactams are primarily eliminated unchanged into the urine *except* drugs in the antistaphylococcal class (metabolized in the liver), and two of the third-generation cephalosporins (cefoperzone and ceftriaxone are eliminated unchanged into the bile).

Adverse Effects

Hypersensitivity. The overall incidence of hypersensitivity reactions is roughly 10% in patients treated with any β-lactam agent. Most of these reactions are mild maculopapular exanthems (skin rash), sometimes accompanied by urticaria, fever, and/or eosinophilia. Other types of hypersensitivity reactions also occur including hemolytic anemia and serum sickness. Fatal anaphylaxis and/or angioedema occur in ~1/100,000 patients treated with any β-lactam agent.

The most important antigenic forms are not β-lactams, but open-ring derivatives that have nonspecifically acylated tissue proteins. Thus, β-lactams sensitize the immune system by functioning as antigenic haptens.

Hypersensivity to one β-lactam agent implies a relatively higher likelihood of a hypersensitive cross-reaction to another β-lactam agent. Between penicillins and cephalosporins, the incidence of cross-reacting hypersensitivity reactions has been estimated to be 10%. Between either of these classes and the carbapenems, the incidence is believed to be higher; between these classes and the monobactams, the incidence appears to be substantially lower.

The incidence of exanthem when administering ampicillin/amoxicillin to patients with Epstein–Barr virus infections (e.g., infectious mononucleosis) approaches 100%. The mechanism of this is not known, but it is not a true hypersensitivity reaction and it is no contraindication to future treatment with any β-lactam agent.

Jarish–Herxheimer Reaction. Severe reactions resembling anaphylactic shock may occur following the administration of β-lactam agents to persons with syphilis. Classically, the reaction occurs within 2 h of treating secondary syphilis with penicillin, but it may occur in other stages of syphilis, with other spirochetal infections (e.g., Lyme), and with agents other than β-lactams. The reaction is due to the release of pyrogens from killed spirochetes, and is not a contraindication to future treatment with the same agent.

Table 2.1.2
β-Lactam Antibiotic Subclasses

Class (examples)	Activity	Comments
Natural penicillin (PCN) (penicillin G, penicillin V)	Streptococci, enterococci, Gram-negative cocci and some bacilli, spirochetes	Despite their introduction six decades ago, these remain the drugs of choice for serious infections (e.g., sepsis, meningitis, pneumonia) caused by susceptible organisms
Aminopenicillins (ampicillin, amoxicillin)	As for PCN, but with broader activity against Gram-negative bacilli	Widely used for otitis, sinusitis, and urinary tract infections
Antistaphylococcal or β-lactamase resistant penicillins (methicillin, nafcillin, oxacillin)	Staphylococcus aureus	Effective against β-lactamase producing bacterial strains, but *not* against methicillin-resistant *S. aureus* (MRSA)
Broad-spectrum or antipseudomonal penicillins (piperacillin, mezlocillin, ticarcillin)	Broad activity against Gram-negative bacilli including pseudomonas, also many anaerobic species and enterococci	Used for infections due to pseudomonas and gastrointestinal flora, and for sepsis in immunocompromised hosts
First-generation cephalosporins (cefazolin, cephalexin)	Staphylococcus and Streptococcus species, some Gram-negative bacteria but not enterococci or gastrointestinal anaerobes	Effective against β-lactamase producing bacterial strains, but not MRSA. Widely used for prophylaxis in surgery.
Second-generation cephalosporins (cefoxitin, cefuroxime, cefotetan)	Compared to first-generation cephalosporins, more Gram-negative activity, less Gram-positive activity, some activity against anaerobic species	Narrow therapeutic niche; prophylaxis in some types of surgical procedures, treatment of pelvic inflammatory disease, mixed aerobe/anaerobe infections

Class	Activity	Notes
Third-generation cephalosporins (ceftriaxone, cefotaxime, ceftazidime, ceftizoxime, cefoperazone)	Broad Gram-negative activity including pseudomonas; little Gram-positive activity	Sometimes the only good therapeutic option for infections due to Gram-negative species; useful for some common sexually transmitted infections (*N. gonorrhea, T. pallidum*) and Lyme disease. The only cephalosporin class that reliably penetrates the blood–brain barrier.
Fourth-generation cephalosporins (cefepime)	More Gram-positive activity than third-generation cephalosporins	Appears to evade destruction by β-lactamases in Gram-negative bacteria by rapidly traversing the periplasm
Monobactams (aztreonam)	Broad Gram-negative activity including pseudomonas; little Gram-positive activity	Least likely β-lactam agent to trigger hypersensitivity reaction in a patient that is hypersensitive to other β-lactams
Carbapenems (imipenem, meropenem)	Broadest Gram-negative and Gram-positive activity of any β-lactam class	Not effective against MRSA, *Xanthomonas* species, or enterococci

Interstitial Nephritis. Impaired renal function with fever, protein-uria, and hematuria is most commonly associated with methicillin, but it can occur with β-lactams from any class.

Platelet Dysfunction. Moxalactam and cefoperazone are associated with platelet dysfunction and bleeding due to the presence of methylthiotetrazole groups.

Drug Interactions

Uncommon.

Mechanisms of Resistance

β-Lactamase Production. β-Lactamase production is the most common mechanism of resistance to β-lactam antibiotics. β-Lactam drugs acylate the active sites of a β-lactamase enzyme in the same way that they acylate the penicillin binding proteins that synthesize the cell wall. However, the acylation of penicillin binding proteins is permanent, while the acylation of a β-lactamase is transient: the enzyme releases the drug as an inactive open-ring form. The net result of this encounter is the destruction of active drug, while enzyme activity is retained.

Many kinds of β-lactamases are known, some with broad nonspecific activity, and some with very specific activity (e.g., oxacillinase, carbenicillinase). They may be chromosomally or plasmid encoded, and constitutively or inducibly expressed. A latent (inducible) capacity to produce β-lactamase can account for the failure of therapy with β-lactam agents when the infecting organism initially appears susceptible.

Gram-positive organisms produce relatively large amounts of β-lactamase because they must secrete the enzyme into an open environment and it must be present in high enough concentration to destroy approaching drug molecules. Gram-negative organisms produce relatively small amounts of β-lactamase because after it is secreted it remains sequestered in the periplasmic space.

Chemical agents are available that specifically inhibit some β-lactamases (e.g. clavulanic acid, sulbactam, and tazobactam. **Fig. 2.1.3**. These agents are β-lactams, but they are not effective as antibiotics. They bind permanently to β-lactamases, and are not released as open ring forms (they exclude water from their binding site; water is necessary to hydrolyze the acyl group and release the open ring form). Treatment with a β-lactamase inhibitor can overcome resistance

β-lactam drugs and β-lactamases

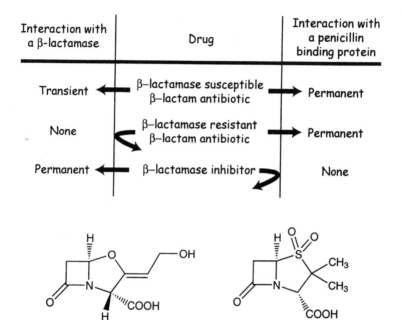

Interaction with a β-lactamase	Drug	Interaction with a penicillin binding protein
Transient ←	β–lactamase susceptible β–lactam antibiotic →	Permanent
None	β–lactamase resistant β–lactam antibiotic →	Permanent
Permanent ←	β–lactamase inhibitor	None

clavulanic acid   sulbactam

tazobactam

Fig. 2.1.3

due to the production of certain types of β-lactamase. β-Lactamase inhibitors are only available in combination with a β-lactamase susceptible agent (amoxacillin and clavulanate—Augmentin; ampicillin and sulbactam—Unasyn; ticarcillin and clavulanate—Timentin; piperacillin and tazobactam—Zosyn).

Porin Deficiency. Porins are specialized channel-forming proteins in the outer membrane of Gram-negative organisms. β-Lactam compounds must penetrate the outer membrane of Gram-negative bacteria to reach their site of action, and the channels formed by porins are necessary in some cases for penetration. Thus, porin deficiency can account for resistance to the action of certain β-lactam agents, most notably cephalosporins and carbapenems.

Methicillin Resistance. Methicillin resistance is due to a mutated form of a penicillin binding protein that results in a low affinity for all β-lactam compounds. Methicillin resistance implies resistance to all β-lactam antibiotics.

Autolysin Deficiency. A deficiency of lytic enzymes gives rise to a "penicillin tolerant" phenotype. Although these organisms may not have the virulence of wild-type organisms, the lack of autolytic enzymes can make the eradication of an infection more difficult.

GLYCOPEPTIDES

Identity

Glycopeptide antibiotics are chemically complex compounds produced by bacteria and purified for therapeutic use **(Fig. 2.1.4)**. They cannot be produced synthetically. They are called glycopeptides because they contain sugar and amino acid residues. Most of the amino acids are not among the 20 amino acids found in proteins, implying that vancomycin is not produced by the translation of a genetic sequence.

More than 100 glycopeptide antibiotics have been identified in nature, but vancomycin is the only one licensed for use in the United States. Teicoplanin is used in Europe. It differs in several respects from vancomycin, most notably in having a lipophilic chain that presumably "anchors" the molecule in lipid membranes. Ristocetin caused bleeding in early trials, and has been deemed too toxic for therapeutic use. For reasons related to this side effect, however, it is

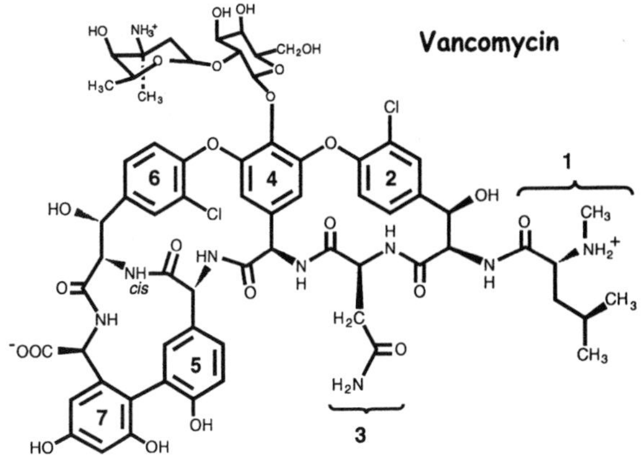

Vancomycin consists of a glucose-vancosamine disaccharide attached to a seven-residue polypeptide chain (residue side chains are numbered). Six of the seven amino acid residues are not among the 20 residues found in proteins, indicating that the polypeptide portion of vancomycin is not genetically encoded, nor is it synthesized on ribosomes.

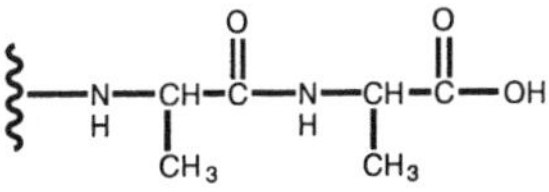

The target of vancomycin action is D-alanyl-D-alanine dipeptide, an intermediate in the synthesis of cell wall peptidoglycan in susceptible bacteria.

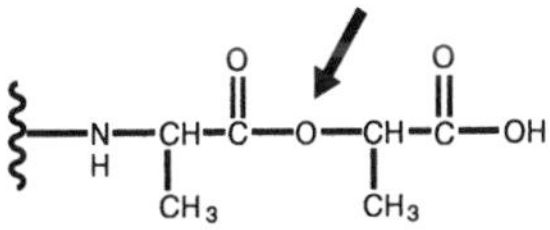

Vancomycin-resistant enterococci (vanA and VanB phenotypes) have replaced D-alanyl-D-alanine with D-alanyl-D-lactate, to which vancomycin cannot bind.

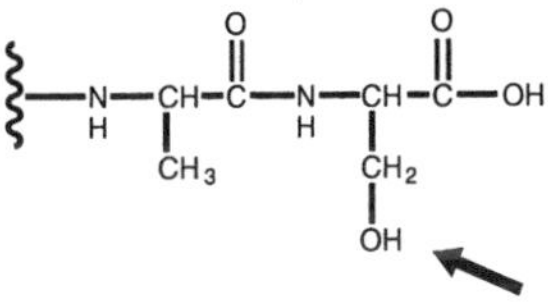

Other vancomycin-resistant bacteria have replaced D-alanyl-D-alanine with D-alanyl-D-serine, to which vancomycin also cannot bind.

Fig. 2.1.4

now used in clinical laboratories for the diagnosis of von Willebrand's disease.

Mechanism of Action

In vancomycin-susceptible organisms, there are two D-alanine residues at the C-terminus of the peptidoglycan precursor prior to crosslinking in the transpeptidation step of peptidoglycan synthesis. During transpeptidation, the terminal D-alanine residue is lost, and the penultimate D-alanine residue is linked to another peptidoglycan precursor. Vancomycin specifically recognizes and binds to the D-alanyl-D-alanine dipeptide, preventing the transpeptidation reaction **(Fig. 2.1.1)**.

Transpeptidation enzymes bind β-lactam antibiotics because β-lactam antibiotics are molecular mimics of the D-alanyl-D-alanine dipeptide. As might be expected, therefore, vancomycin has some affinity for β-lactam antibiotics, although its affinity is too low to cause any significant drug–drug interaction.

Activity

Glycopeptide antibiotics are active only against Gram-positive organisms whose peptidoglycan precursors have terminal D-alanyl-D-alanine dipeptides. Vancomycin is excluded from its site of action by the outer membrane of Gram-negative bacteria, and the peptidoglycan precursors of some pathologically significant Gram-positive bacteria terminate with D-alanyl-D-serine dipeptides or D-alanyl-D-lactate depsipeptides that are not recognized by vancomycin **(Fig. 2.1.4)**. Vancomycin is commonly used against staphylococci, streptococci, and enterococci when attempting to overcome resistance or circumvent hypersensitivity reactions to other agents.

Administration, Metabolism, and Elimination

Vancomycin is administered orally only in the treatment of antibiotic-induced colitis because it is not absorbed from the gastrointestinal tract. In all other cases, it is administered intravenously. It is eliminated unchanged in the urine.

Compared to most other antibiotics, vancomycin has a narrow therapeutic index. This necessitates diligent pharmacokinetic monitoring of blood levels during therapy. Although vancomycin is relatively inexpensive, the costs of intravenous administration and monitoring make the cost of vancomycin therapy relatively high.

Adverse Effects

Auditory nerve damage with tinnitus, dysequilibrium, and hearing loss is common with higher blood levels. This damage is particularly serious because it is usually irreversible.

Early impure preparations were associated with nephrotoxicity, but this is not a significant problem with current preparations.

Rapid intravenous infusion can cause thrombophlebitis and/or the "red man syndrome" with facial flushing, hypotension, and shock due to the stimulation of histamine release. The symptoms resolve quickly when the infusion is halted, and usually do not recur if the infusion is resumed at a slower rate. Thus, it is not a hypersensitivity reaction, and is not a contraindication to further therapy with vancomycin.

Drug Interactions

None of clinical significance.

Mechanisms of Resistance

There are at least two explanations for the slow emergence of vancomycin resistance. First, it binds to the substrate of the transglycosylation/transpeptidation reactions, rather than to the enzymes catalyzing these reactions. Because this substrate is the result of a complex multicomponent biosynthetic pathway, it is unlikely that resistance could arise from a simple single-site mutation. Second, vancomycin must be administered intravenously. This relegated it to relatively infrequent use in hospitalized patients and reduced both the selective pressure for resistance and the likelihood of suboptimal dosing. Vancomycin was used for several decades under the assumption that staphylococci, streptococci, and enterococci were uniformly susceptible. Since 1989, however, enterococci are being isolated in increasing numbers with a plasmid-encoded set of enzymes that provide for peptidoglycan synthesis by an inducible alternative path **(Fig 2.1.4)**. When both vancomycin and teicoplanin induce this path, the resistance phenotype is designated vanA. When vancomycin but not teicoplanin induces this path, the phenotype is designated vanB. Other less common inducible resistance phenotypes also exist, as does constitutive resistance (e.g., *Lactobacillus spp.*).

It is likely that the heavy use of avoparcin, a closely related glycopeptide antibiotic, as a growth promoting additive to animal feed in Europe was a major factor in the emergence of vancomycin resistance.

The incidence of vancomycin-resistant enterococci now exceeds 50% of all enterococcal infections in many hospitals, making this a major public health problem.

Strains of methicillin-resistant *S. aureus* have been isolated that exhibit an intermediate level of susceptibility to vancomycin. Morphologically, these organisms exhibit exceptionally thick cell walls, and the clinical significance of this reduced susceptibility is not clear at this time.

2.2 Antifolate Agents (Table 2.2)

Identity

Sulfonamides are simple synthetic compounds related to *p*-aminobenzoic acid **(Fig. 2.2)**. Dapsone is so named because it is a symmetric di-anilino-para-sulfone. Trimethoprim and pyrimethamine do not contain sulfur.

Mechanism of Action

Many bacteria absorb *p*-aminobenzoate, convert it into dihydrofolate and tetrahydrofolate, and then ultimately use it to synthesize purines for nucleic acid **(Fig. 2.2)**. By virtue of their chemical resemblance to *p*-aminobenzoate, sulfonamides inhibit the synthesis of folates. In contrast, human metabolism relies on dietary folates, and some bacteria have developed means to absorb preformed folates in their environment. Thus, they are unaffected by the action of sulfonamides.

Trimethoprim and pyrimethamine inhibit the conversion of dihydrofolate to tetrahydrofolate by bacterial forms of dihydrofolate reductase. The human form of dihydrofolate reductase is relatively insensitive to inhibition by these drugs (although it is highly sensitive to inhibition by the anticancer agent methotrexate).

Sulfonamides and trimethoprim are commonly used in combination because (a) they inhibit two different reactions on the same metabolic pathway and thus exhibit synergistic activity, and (b) the combination reduces the likelihood that resistance will develop.

Activity

Many organisms once susceptible are now resistant to sulfonamides, often due to single-step mutations in the target enzyme. However, useful activity still includes many Gram-positive and Gram-negative

Table 2.2
Currently Marketed Antifolate Antibiotics

Generic name	Oral	IV	IM	Top	Trade names
Mafenide				X	Sulfamylon
Sulfabenzamide				X	Gyne-Sulf,[a] Triple-sulfa,[a] Trysul,[a] Sultrin,[a] Dayto[a]
Sulfacetamide				X	Ak-Cide, Vasosulf, Vasocidin, Triple-sulfa,[a] Blephamide, Bleph-10 Dayto,[a] Cetapred, Trysul,[a] Bleph, Predsulfair, Sulf-10, Sulfac, Sulf, Metimyd, Fml, Fml-S, Klaron, Gyne-Sulf,[a] Ocusulf, Isopto, Sulster, Sultrin[a]
Sulfacytine	X				Renoquid
Sulfadiazine	X				Triple-sulfa[a]
Sulfadoxine	X				Fansidar[a]
Sulfamerazine	X				Triple-sulfa[a]
Sulfamethazine	X				Triple-sulfa[a]
Sulfamethizole	X				Urobiotic-250[a]
Sulfamethoxazole	X	X			Bethaprim,[a] Bactrim,[a] Sulfameth/Trimeth,[a] Smz-Tmp,[a] Sulfameth,[a] Sulfamethoxozole,[a] Cotrim,[a] Sulfatrim,[a] Sultrex,[a] Gantanol, Septra,[a] Smx,[a] Bacter-Aid,[a] Trimeth,[a] Trimethoprim[a]
Sulfanilamide				X	Avc
Sulfasalazine	X				Azulfidine
Sulfathiazole				X	Dayto,[a] Gyne-Sulf,[a] Triple-sulfa,[a] Trysul,[a] Sultrin*
Sulfisoxazole	X				Eryzole,[a] E, Azo,[a] Ery, Pediazole,[a] Pediagen,[a] Erythro-Sul,[a] Truxazole, Gantrisin
Trimethoprim	X	X		X	Sulfameth,[a] Polytrim,[a] Sulfatrim,[a] Sulfamethoxozole,[a] Bactrim,[a] Proloprim, Smz,[a] Septra,[a] Smz-Tmp,[a] Bethaprim,[a] Sultrex,[a] Smx,[a] Bacter-Aid,[a] Sulfamethoxazole, Cotrim,[a] Trimeth,[a] Trimethoprim/, Trimpex, Sulfameth/Trimeth[a]

[a]Multicomponent product

O, oral; IV, intravenous; IM, intramuscular; T, topical, including preparations applied to skin, eyes, and ears

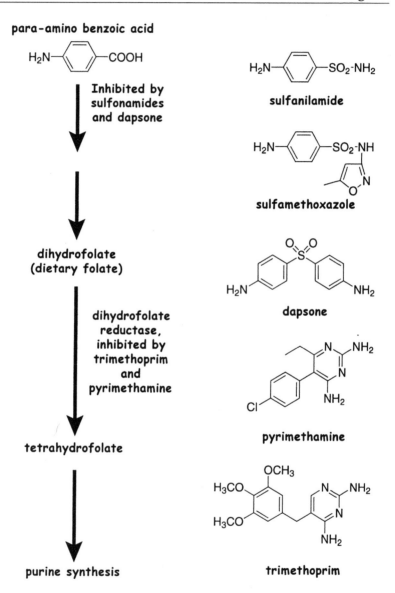

Fig. 2.2

organisms as well as actinomyces, chlamydia, malaria, pneumocystis, and toxoplasma. Trimethoprim has been used as a single agent for the treatment of urinary tract infections and traveler's diarrhea, but is much more widely used in a fixed combination with sulfamethoxazole to achieve synergistic activity. Pyrimethamine is combined with sulfadoxine for use against chloroquine-resistant malaria, and with dapsone for use against pneumocystis. Dapsone also has an important role in the treatment of leprosy.

Administration, Metabolism, and Elimination

Most drugs in this class are well absorbed from the gastrointestinal tract and distribute well into most tissues including the central nervous system (CNS). Most are eliminated unchanged into the urine, although some undergo modification in the liver before elimination into the urine. The only significant exception is sulfasalazine, which is poorly absorbed from the gastrointestinal tract. This drug passes through to the colon where it is metabolized by bacterial enzymes into sulfapyridine and 5-amino-salicylic acid. The latter has local anti-inflammatory effects and most likely accounts for the beneficial effects of sulfasalazine in inflammatory bowel disease.

The rate at which sulfonamides are eliminated in the urine varies according to the extent to which they are protein bound. Short-acting sulfonamides with half-lives of <20 h are used primarily for urinary tract infections because their rapid elimination results in high urinary concentrations. Sulfamethoxazole is frequently combined with trimethoprim (cotrimoxazole) because they have similar and relatively slow rates of elimination. This helps maintain optimal relative concentrations in the blood. Sulfadoxine has a half life of 100–200 h, and can therefore be used for once-per-week dosing.

Adverse Effect

Hypersensivity reactions are common. Most often these reactions are minor exanthems, but a variety of more severe reactions are all known to occur. Long-acting forms are associated with a severe life-threatening hypersensivity reaction known as the Stevens–Johnson syndrome, particularly in children.

Sulfonamides can cause hemolysis in glucose 6-phosphate dehydrogenase (G6PD) deficient patients, and rapidly eliminated forms can cause crystalluria. This is best avoided by maintaining alkaline urine and high output.

Drug Interactions

Sulfonamides displace many other drugs from plasma proteins, acutely raising their potency, but subacutely increasing their rate of elimination. These include warfarin, methotrexate, oral contraceptives, oral hypoglycemic agents, thiazide diuretics, and phenytoin. Sulfonamide kinetics may be altered when they are displaced from protein binding sites by common antiinflammatory drugs such as salicylates, indomethacin, and phenylbutazone.

Mechanisms of Resistance

Resistance to sulfonamides and trimethoprim is widespread and operates by various mechanisms (chromosomal mutation in the target enzyme, plasmid-mediated acquisition of alternative forms of the target enzymes, reduced permeability of the cell membrane, and altered means of *p*-aminobenzoic acid [PABA] utilization).

2.3. Aminoglycosides / Aminocyclitols (Table 2.3)

Identity (Fig. 2.3)

Streptomycin, kanamycin, and tobramycin are single-component natural products (purified from different species of *Streptomyces*). Neomycin and gentamicin are mixtures of closely related naturally occurring compounds. Amikacin and netilmicin are semisynthetic derivatives of naturally occurring compounds. The "-micins" and "-mycins" are derived from different organisms. (*Note:* there are no drugs with the suffix "-myosin.")

Mechanism of Action.

Aminoglycosides penetrate bacterial cell membranes by means of an energy-dependent carrier mechanism. Once in the bacterial cell, they bind to both subunits of the bacterial ribosome, interfering with their assembly, and causing mRNA to be misread. Because the antibacterial activity of aminoglycosides seems out of proportion to its ability to interfere with protein synthesis, it is believed they also have other sites or mechanisms of action.

Activity

Aminoglycosides are primarily used against Gram-negative bacteria, although they are also used against Gram-positive bacteria in

Table 2.3
Currently Marketed Aminoglycoside Antibiotics

Generic name	O	IV	IM	T	Trade names
Amikacin		X	X		Amikin
Gentamicin		X	X	X	Garamycin, Gentasol, Gentak, Gentagen, Gentafair, Genoptic, Gentacidin
Kanamycin	X	X	X		Kantrex
Neomycin	X		X	X	Duomycin-Hc,[a] Dexasporin,[a] Dexacidin,[a] Cortomycin,[a] Cortisporin,[a] Bio-Cot,[a] Bacitracin,[a] Gatol,[a] Neoptic,[a] Otimar,[a] Oticin,[a] Poly-Pred,[a] Octicair,[a] Npd,[a] Maxitrol,[a] Neosporin,[a] Methadex,[a] Neopolydex,[a] Neodecadron, Neocin, Neocidin,[a] Neo-Fradin, Neomycin, Polymycin,[a] Ak-Trol,[a] Genosporin,[a] Alba[a]
Paromomycin	X				Humatin
Streptomycin			X		
Tobramycin		X	X	X	Aktob, Tobi, Tobradex, Tobrasol, Tobrex, Tomycine, Nebcin

[a]Multicomponent product

O, oral; IV, intravenous; IM, intramuscular; T, topical, including preparations applied to skin, eyes, and ears

33

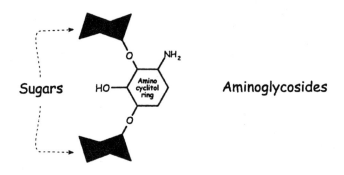

Fig. 2.3

conjunction with cell wall active agents. They have important roles in the treatment of tularemia, bubonic plague, and brucella infections. Some drugs in this class also have activity against mycobacteria. Paromomycin is administered orally for the treatment of intestinal parasitic infections, and parenterally for leishmaniasis.

Aminoglycosides are inactive in acidic or hypoxic environments (e.g., abscess). In some cases (e.g., pseudomonas), aminoglycosides appear to have a significant "post-antibiotic effect". They are often used to suppress the emergence of resistance to other drugs being administered concomitantly, although in most cases this indication is speculative.

Administration, Metabolism, and Elimination

Drugs in this class are not absorbed from the gastrointestinal tract and they penetrate poorly outside the vascular and interstitial compartments. They are eliminated unchanged into the urine.

Most dosing strategies involve a loading dose that is not corrected for renal function impairment, followed by maintenance doses that are adjusted according to renal function. They have a relatively low therapeutic index, necessitating diligent pharmacokinetic monitoring of blood levels during therapy. Exceeding either the recommended peak or trough levels is associated with increased likelihood of toxicity. The costs of intravenous administration and monitoring make the cost of aminoglycoside therapy relatively high.

Adverse Effects

A mild degree of nonoliguric renal failure is common during therapy, but usually reversible. The risk is related to blood levels above target ranges, advanced age, female gender, liver disease, and hypotension.

Damage to both auditory and vestibular branches of cranial nerve VIII is also common, and is usually of greater consequence because it is irreversible.

Aminoglycosides can cause temporary neuromuscular paralysis. This occurs rarely, but can be serious.

Drug Interactions.

The risk of neuromuscular paralysis is higher in combination with other agents acting on the neuromuscular junction, e.g., succinylcholine.

Mechanisms of Resistance

Enzymatic conjugation is the most common mechanism of resistance. Plasmid-mediated conjugating enzymes are of three types: acetylation, adenylation, and phosphorylation. Note that bacteria conjugate and inactivate aminoglycosides, whereas humans do not alter these drugs prior to elimination in the urine. Different plasmids bearing enzymes with specificities for different aminoglycosides predominate in different hospitals.

There are a large number of enzymes that inactivate gentamicin, but somewhat fewer that inactivate amikacin. This has led to a policy of holding amikacin "in reserve," for use only in cases of proven gentamicin resistance, or when gentamicin resistance has become prevalent. These policies alter the prevalence of different plasmid-encoded enzymes by altering selective pressure.

Bacteria may also resist aminoglycosides by inactivating their influx mechanism. This is a serious problem in some hospitals, but rare in most.

2.4 Antiribosomal Agents (Table 2.4 and Fig. 2.4)

30S AGENTS: TETRACYCLINE

Identity **(Fig. 2.4.1)**

Mechanism of Action

Tetracyclines reversibly bind to the 30S subunit of the bacterial ribosome and inhibit protein synthesis (by interfering with aminoacyl-

Table 2.4
Currently Marketed Antiribosomal Antibiotics

Subclass	Generic name	O	IV	IM	T	Trade names
30S subunit target (tetracyclines)	Tetracycline	X	X		X	Actisite, Achromycin, Brodspec, Sumycin, Tetra
	Demeclocycline	X				Declomycin
	Doxycycline	X	X			Vibramycin, Periostat, Doxychel, Atridox, Doryx, Bio-Tab, Doxal, Doxy-Cap, Vibra-Tabs, Doxy-Tabs, Monodox
	Minocycline	X	X			Vectrin, Dynacin, Minocin
	Oxytetracycline	X	X	X	X	Urobiotic-250,[a] Terramycin,[a] Geomycin
30S subunit target (other)	Spectinomycin			X		Trobicin
50S subunit target (macrolides)	Azithromycin	X	X			Zithromax
	Clarithromycin	X				Biaxin
	Dirithromycin	X				Dynabac
	Erythromicin	X			X	Erythromicin, Akne-Mycin, Erythra, Emgel, Ergel, Ery-C, Erytab, Erymax, E-Mycin, Romycin, PCE
	Erythromycin estolate	X				Ilosone
	Erythromycin Ethylsuccinate	X				Pediazole,[a] Ees,[a] Pediagen,[a] Erythro-Sul,[a] Eryzole,[a] Eryped
	Erythromycin Lactobionate		X			Erythrocin[a]
	Erythromycin stearate	X				Erythrocin,[a] Erythrocot
	Troleandomycin	X				Tao

50S subunit target (ketolides)		O	IV	IM	T	
	Telithromycin	X				Ketek
50S subunit target (other)	Chloramphenicol	X	X		X	Chloroptic, Chloromycetin
	Clindamycin	X	X	X	X	Cleocin, Clinda-Derm, Clindamylin
	Lincomycin	X	X	X	X	Bactramycin, Lincocin, Lincoject
(oxazolidinones)	Linezolid	X	X		X	Zyvox
(streptogramins)	Dalfopristin		X		X	Synercid[a]
	Quinupristin		X		X	Synercid[a]

[a]Multicomponent product

O, oral; IV, intravenous; IM, intramuscular; T, topical, including preparations applied to skin, eyes, and ears.

Antiribosomal agents

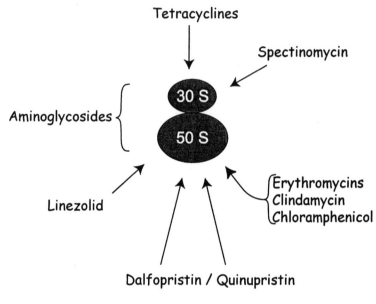

Fig. 2.4

tRNA binding). Their ability to penetrate the outer membrane of Gram-negative bacteria relies on porins. Penetration of the inner membrane is an energy-dependent carrier-mediated process.

Activity

Many organisms once susceptible are now resistant to tetracyclines, but useful activity remains among many Gram-positive and Gram-negative organisms. They exhibit important activity against *Rickettsia, Mycoplasma, Chlamydia,* and spirochetes including *Borrelia.* They are also used prophylactically against malaria and travelers' diarrhea.

Administration, Metabolism, and Elimination

The absorption of tetracyclines from the gastrointestinal tract is carrier mediated, and the capacity of this carrier is readily saturated. As a consequence, their bioavailability decreases with increasing dose.

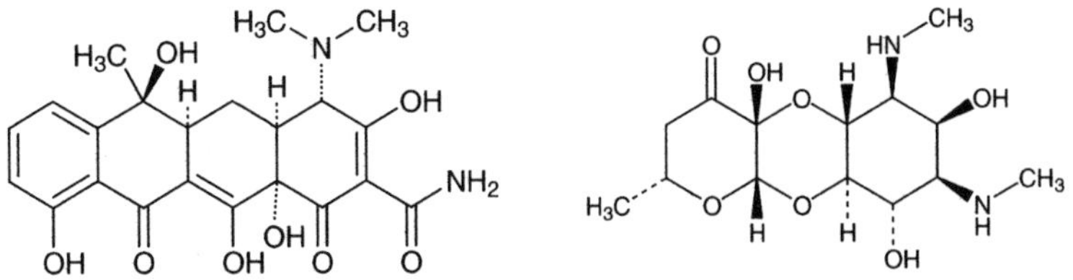

Tetracycline   Spectinomycin

Fig. 2.4.1

They exhibit complex elimination kinetics because of their propensity to bind divalent cations (dairy products, antacids, bone, tooth enamel), and their tendency to be transported via carriers (elimination into saliva, tears, respiratory secretions, as well as urine and bile).

Adverse Effects

Photosensitivity is of particular importance because these agents tend to be useful when travelling to areas where sun exposure is relatively high. They are contraindicated in pregnancy because their propensity to bind divalent cations (e.g., calcium) results in a discoloration of developing teeth and a depression of bone growth in children. They tend to form nephrotoxic degradation products on long storage (Fanconi's syndrome).

Drug Interactions.

Decreased absorption with antacids containing calcium and magnesium (i.e., divalent cations).

Mechanisms of Resistance

Bacteria can resist the action of tetracyclines by losing their influx pump, or by acquiring a plasmid that encodes for an efflux pump.

30S AGENTS: SPECTINOMYCIN

Spectinomycin is a tricyclic compound often misleadingly grouped with the aminoglycosides, but its structure **(Fig. 2.4.1)**, mechanism of action, and spectrum of activity all differ markedly from the aminoglycosides. It binds to the 30S subunit of the bacterial ribosome, This drug has a single indication: the treatment of gonorrhea in persons for whom other recommended treatments are not safe or available, and for whom a single intramuscular injection is advantageous.

50S AGENTS: MACROLIDES

Identity

Macrolides consist of a large 14- or 15-membered ring to which two sugar residues are attached.

Mechanism of Action

Macrolides have a dual mechanism of action. They bind to 50S subunit of bacterial ribosome and inhibit protein synthesis by inhibiting transpeptidation and translocation. This binding site overlaps with that of clindamycin and chloramphenicol. They also inhibit the formation of the 50S ribosomal subunit. Delays inherent in the formation of new 50S particles account for prolonged postantibiotic effects (*see* Section 1.4).

Activity

They exhibit broad Gram-positive and Gram-negative activity, with important activity against *Legionella*, mycoplasma, *Chlamydia*, *Rickettsia*, *Helicobacter*, spirochetes, and anaerobes. Spiramycin appears to have some activity against *Cryptosporidium* and *Toxoplasma*. Their antimicrobial activity increases markedly as environmental pH increases from 5.5 to 8.5.

Administration, Metabolism, and Elimination

Tissue half-lives are much longer than half-lives in blood, and tissue concentrations may be orders of magnitude higher than blood concentration. For this reason, dosing intervals and duration of action are usually much longer than the serum half-lives (erythromycin, < 2 h; clarithromycin, 5-7 h; azithromycin, 35–40 h).

Erythromycin is degraded by stomach acid (the ester linkage in the ring is acid-labile), and causes phlebitis when administered intravenously [due to the basic $N(CH_3)_2$ group on one of its sugars]. For oral administration, acid-stable stearate, estolate, and ethylsuccinate conjugates are available. For intravenous administration, gluceptate and lactobionate salts are more soluble and less likely to cause phlebitis.

Adverse Effects

Gastrointestinal disturbance is common with all forms of erythromycin, but it is less common or less severe with clarithromycin and azithromycin. The cause of this disturbance is related to the stimulation of gut receptors for motilin, a hormone regulating gut motility.

Drug Interactions

Macrolides decrease hepatic metabolism and increase the pharmacological effects of many drugs (including warfarin, prednisone, theophyilline, cyclosporin, carbamazepine, digoxin). Macrolides antagonize the action of chloramphenicol and clindamycin due to their overlapping binding sites on the ribosome.

Mechanisms of Resistance

Bacteria resist macrolide action by a variety of mechanisms including reduced permeability, active efflux, enzymatic digestion, and chromosomal mutations that alter protein or RNA in the ribosomal binding site. In addition to these mechanisms, there is a gene that confers macrolide resistance by methylating ribosomal RNA. The presence of this gene is associated with resistance to clindamycin and streptogramins as well as both macrolides and ketolides.

50S AGENTS: KETOLIDES

With the introduction of telithromycin, ketolides become the newest class of antimicrobial drugs available in the United States. Ketolides are closely related to macrolides in structure **(Fig. 2.4.2)**, and share a similar dual mechanism of action. However, telithromycin is active against many organisms that are resistant to erythromycin, although it may not be effective against some species in which macrolide resistance is due to methylated ribosomal RNA.

50S AGENTS: CHLORAMPHENICOL

Identity **(Fig. 2.4.3)**

Chloramphenicol is the least expensive and most widely available antimicrobial agent in underdeveloped countries.

Mechanism of Action.

Chloramphenicol penetrates the microbial membrane by an energy-dependent influx mechanism and binds to the 50S subunit of bacterial ribosomes, inhibiting protein synthesis. Its binding site overlaps that of erythromycin and clindamycin.

Activity

Chloramphenicol exhibits diverse activity against Gram-negative and Gram-positive organisms, especially anaerobes. It has especially

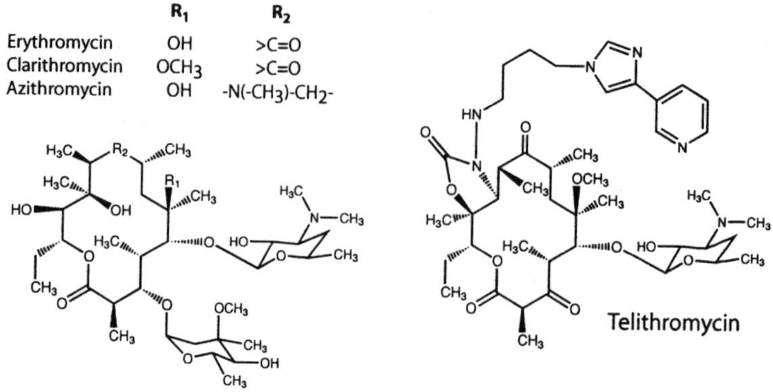
R1 R2
Erythromycin OH >C=O
Clarithromycin OCH3 >C=O
Azithromycin OH -N(-CH3)-CH2-
Telithromycin

Fig. 2.4.2

important activity against rickettsia, mycoplasma, and spirochetes, and is also used for the treatment of deep abscesses, Typhoid Fever, Rocky Mountain Spotted Fever, and infections due to vancomycin-resistant enterococci.

Administration, Metabolism, and Elimination

The bioavailability of chloramphenicol is high, and it readily penetrates all body tissues, as well as abscess cavities. It is inactivated by conjugation in the liver.

Adverse Effects.

Chloramphenicol reliably causes reversible dose-related bone marrow suppression, probably due to interference with protein synthesis by mitochondrial ribosomes.

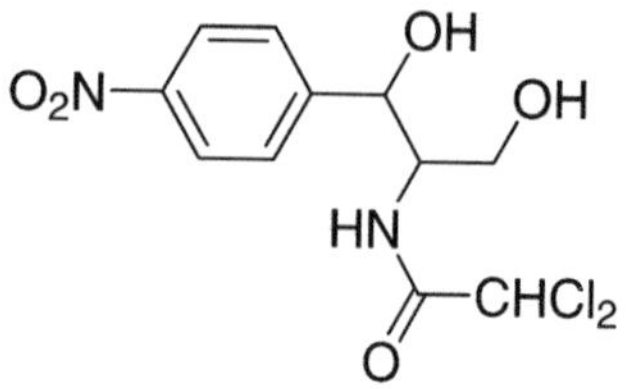
O2N
OH
OH
HN
CHCl2
O

Chloramphenicol

Fig. 2.4.3

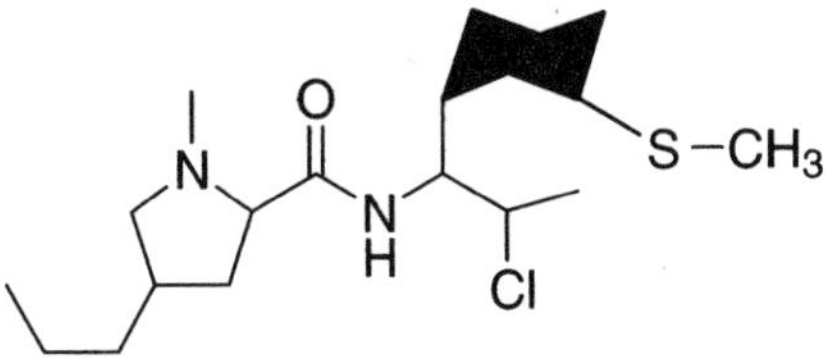

Fig. 2.4.4

In contrast, it also causes irreversible idiosyncratic aplastic anemia that is fatal without bone marrow transplant. Most of these reactions follow oral administration, suggesting that a metabolic product of intestinal bacteria may be responsible. Incidence is between 1/25,000 and 1/40,000 patients.

Drug Interactions

Chloramphenicol inhibits the metabolism of many other drugs by microsomal enzymes, thereby prolonging the action of oral hypoglycemic agents, phenytoin, cyclophosphamide, and warfarin. It antagonizes the action of macrolides and clindamycin due to their overlapping binding sites on the ribosome.

Mechanisms of Resistance.

Bacteria may resist the action of chloramphenicol by shutting down their influx mechanism, or by acquiring a plasmid encoding for chloramphenicol acetyltransferase.

50S AGENTS: CLINDAMYCIN

Identity **(Fig. 2.4.4)**

Mechanism of Action

Clindamycin binds to the 50S subunit of bacterial ribosomes and inhibits protein synthesis. Its binding site overlaps that of erythromycin and chloramphenicol.

Activity

Clindamycin has important activity against Gram-positive and Gram-negative anaerobes, *Babesia,* and *Toxoplasma.* Occasionally, it is also used against methicillin-resistant *S. aureus,* and other Gram-positive aerobes.

Administration, Metabolism, and Elimination

Clindamycin is well absorbed, metabolized in the liver to the
N-demethyl form, and eliminated into the bile. *N*-demethyl clindamycin has more activity than its parent compound, and has major
effects on bowel flora. For intravenous administration, clindamycin
is administered as the phosphate ester which is rapidly hydrolyzed in
vivo. A tendency to concentrate in bone makes clindamycin a favored
agent for the treatment of osteomyelitis.

Adverse Effects

Clindamycin therapy is frequently accompanied by diarrhea,
but mild and uncomplicated diarrhea (antibiotic-associated diarrhea) must be distinguished from pseudomembranous or antibiotic-
associated colitis (AAC), a serious and even life-threatening condition.
AAC is caused by toxins from *C. difficile,* which overgrows the colonic
flora during clindamycin therapy. The incidence is reported to vary
from 1/10 to 1/10,000 in different studies. Classically, AAC is caused
by clindamycin, but may also be caused by any antibiotic that alters
the normal colonic bacterial flora. It is treated by discontinuing the
precipitating antibiotic, and the oral administration of vancomycin
or metronidazole.

Drug Interactions

Clindamycin antagonizes the action of macrolides and chloramphenicol due to their overlapping binding sites on the ribosome. It
may prolong the action of neuromuscular blocking agents.

Mechanisms of Resistance

Resistance is most commonly due to altered ribosomal proteins and
ribosomal RNA. These alterations typically exhibit cross-resistance
to erythromycin and chloramphenicol.

50S AGENTS: OXAZOLIDINONES

Identity (**Fig. 2.4.5**)

Mechanism of Action

Oxazolidinones bind to the 50S subunit of the bacterial ribosome
and inhibit protein synthesis by preventing the initiation of mRNA
translation.

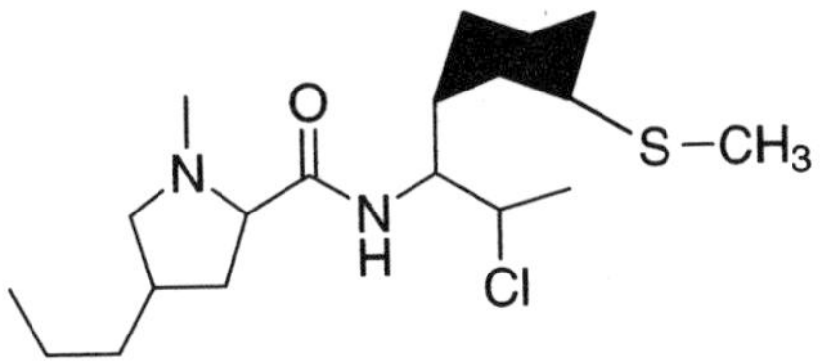

Clindamycin

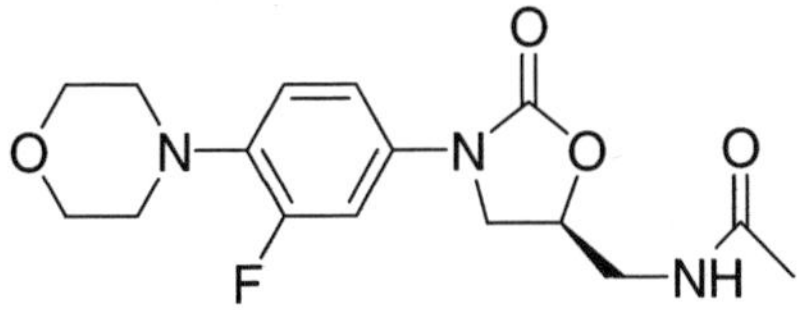

Fig. 2.4.5

Activity

This class of antibiotics was developed to target vancomycin-resistant enterococci, methicillin-resistant *S. aureus*, and drug resistant *S. pneumoniae*.

Administration, Metabolism, and Elimination

Well absorbed orally; oral administration achieves the same blood levels as intravenous administration.

Adverse Effects

Information about safety profile is limited, but various forms of myelo-suppression appear to be common with prolonged administration.

Drug Interactions

Linezolid is an inhibitor of monoamine oxidase and may therefore elevate blood pressure in persons taking pseudoephedrine or phenylpropanolamine.

Mechanisms of Resistance

Gram positive resistance due to mutations in ribosomal RNA have been reported. Gram-negative bacteria appear to have an active efflux mechanism.

50S AGENTS: STREPTOGRAMINS

Identity **(Fig. 2.4.6)**

Streptogramins are produced in nature as synergistic pairs. Naturally occurring pristinamycin/virginiamycin is used in Europe. Quinupristin and dalfopristin comprise a pair of semisynthetic derivatives marketed in the United States as Synercid.

Mechanism of Action

Streptogramins bind to two different sites on the 50S subunit of the bacterial ribosome, and inhibit protein synthesis at two different

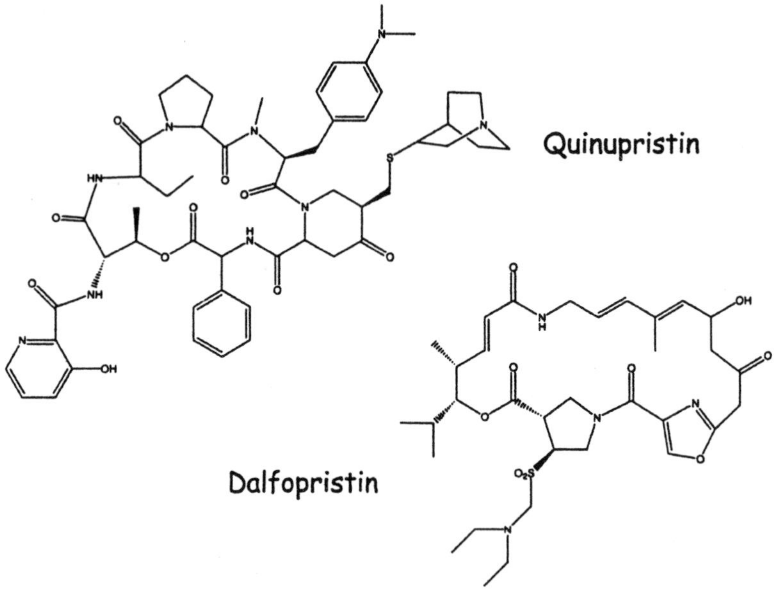

Fig. 2.4.6

stages, thereby exerting strongly synergistic activity. Binding of quinupristin increases the affinity of dalfopristin for its binding site, and their combined action is irreversible.

Activity

Streptogramins are active against *E. faecium* (including vancomycin-resistant strains), but it is important to note that they are not active against *E. faecalis*. They may also be used against some staphylococcal and streptococcal infections.

Administration, Metabolism, and Elimination

These agents require intravenous administration.

Adverse Effects

Severe arthralgias and myalgias are common.

Drug Interactions

Inhibits a widely used hepatic P450 enzyme (CYP 3A4), and is therefore likely to interact with many other drugs.

Table 2.5
Currently Marketed Topoisomerase Inhibitors

Generic name	O	IV	IM	T	Trade names
Alatrofloxacin		X			Trovan
Cinoxacin	X				Cinobac
Ciprofloxacin	X	X		X	Cipro, Ciloxan
Enoxacin	X				Penetrex
Gatifloxacin	X	X			Tequin
*Grepafloxacin	X				Raxar
Levofloxacin	X	X			Levaquin
Lomefloxacin	X				Maxaquin
Moxifloxacin	X				Avelox
Norfloxacin	X			X	Noroxin, Chibroxin
Ofloxacin	X	X		X	Floxin, Ocuflox
Sparfloxacin	X				Zagam
Trovafloxacin	X				Trovana

O, oral; IV, intravenous; IM, intramuscular; T, topical, including preparations applied to skin, eyes, and ears
* Withdrawn

Mechanisms of Resistance

Cross-resistance with erythromycin/clindamycin, intracellular degradation, and efflux mechanisms have been reported. The occurrence of primary resistance to streptogramins as a class has been linked to the use of virginiamycin as an animal growth promoter in Europe.

2.5 Topoisomerase Inhibitors (Quinolones, Table 2.1.5)

Identity **(Fig. 2.5)**

The quinolones are chemically related to nalidixic acid, an antimicrobial introduced more than 40 y ago for urinary tract infections. The key modification that led to more potent agents was the addition of a fluorine atom, so they are also known as fluoroquinolones.

Purification of the "levo-" stereoisomer of ofloxacin from a racemic mixture of levo and the inactive "dextro-" form yields levofloxacin—a preparation with twice the antimicrobial potency of ofloxacin. Alatrofloxacin is a prodrug form of trovafloxacin intended for intravenous administration.

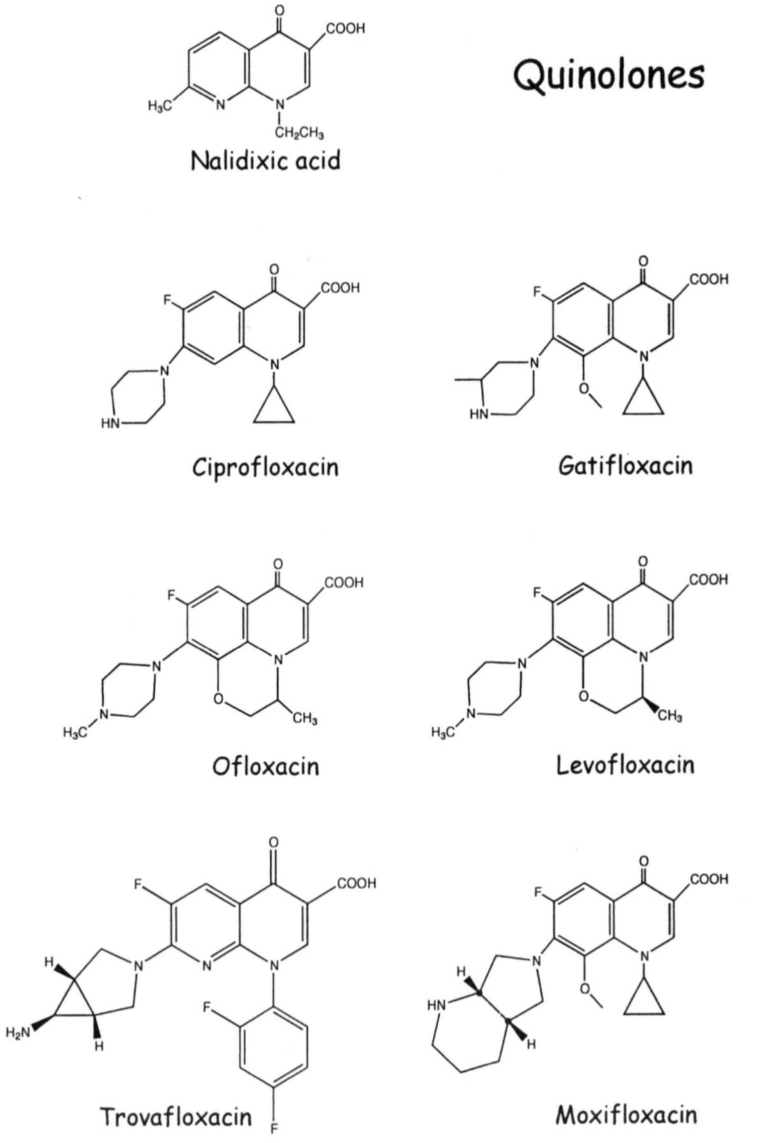

Quinolones

Nalidixic acid

Ciprofloxacin

Gatifloxacin

Ofloxacin

Levofloxacin

Trovafloxacin

Moxifloxacin

Fig. 2.5

Mechanism of Action

Quinolones inhibit DNA synthesis by inhibiting two topoisomerases that are essential to bacterial replication: DNA gyrase, which induces supercoiling of the chromosome, and topoisomerase IV, which helps divide replicated chromosomes.

Activity

Quinolones exhibit broad activity against Gram-negative and Gram-positive organisms, although it is highly variable among different agents in this class. Some of these antibiotics exhibit important activity against pseudomonas, xanthomonas, chlamydia, and some mycobacteria.

Administration, Metabolism, and Elimination

Althought their bioavailability is generally good, some agents (nalidixic acid, norfloxacin) achieve therapeutic concentrations only in the urine.

Adverse Effects

Quinolones are generally well tolerated, but relatively contraindicated in children due to possible effects on mineralization of cartilage.

Drug Interactions

Their absorption from the gastrointestinal tract is hindered by antacids and iron/zinc-containing multivitamins. They also reduce the elimination of theophylline

Mechanisms of Resistance

Resistant bacteria often have mutations in the target enzyme, but more complex resistance mechanisms also appear to be present.

2.6 Miscellaneous Agents (Table 2.6)

METRONIDAZOLE

Identity (**Fig. 2.6.1**)

Mechanism of Action

Under anaerobic conditions, metronidazole is activated by a bacterial enzyme that reduces (adds an electron to) the NO_2 group. This has two consequences. First, it converts the drug into a highly reactive free radical that damages various proteins and nucleic acids by forming chemical adducts. This traps converted drug in the cell, so there

Table 2.6
Miscellaneous Currently Marketed Antibiotics

Generic name	O	IV	IM	T	Trade names
Bacitracin			X	X	Neosporin,[a] Neocin,[a] Baciim, Polysporin,[a] Cortomycin,[a] Cortisporin,[a] Neocidin,[a] Polycidin,[a] Neomycin,[a] Ocumycin,[a] Triple-antibiotic,[a] Polymycin,[a] Polytracin,[a] Polycin[a]
Gramicidin				X	Neosporin,[a] Triple-antibiotic,[a] Alba,[a] Neomycin,[a] Neocin,[a] Polymycin,[a] Neoptic,[a] Neocidin[a]
Metronidazole	X	X		X	Flagyl, Noritate, Metrocream, Metrogel, Metron
Mupirocin				X	Bactroban
Polymyxin		X	X	X	Triple-antibiotic,[a] Cortisporin,[a] Duomycin-Hc,[a] Dexacidin,[a] Cortomycin,[a] Gatol,[a] Terramycin,[a] Genosporin,[a] Dexasporin,[a] Oticin,[a] Poly-Pred,[a] Otimar,[a] Methadex,[a] Otobiotic, Polymixin, Npd,[a] Neo,[a] Neopolydex,[a] Polytrim,[a] Alba,[a] Neoptic,[a] Bio-Cot,[a] Polycin,[a] Bacitracin,[a] Polymycin,[a] Neomycin,[a] Neocin,[a] Polysporin,[a] Neocidin,[a] Maxitrol,[a] Neosporin,[a] Polytracin,[a] Octicair,[a] Polycidin,[a] Ak-Trol,[a] Ocumycin[a]

[a]Multicomponent product
O, oral; IV, intravenous; IM, intramuscular; T, topical, including preparations applied to skin, eyes, and ears

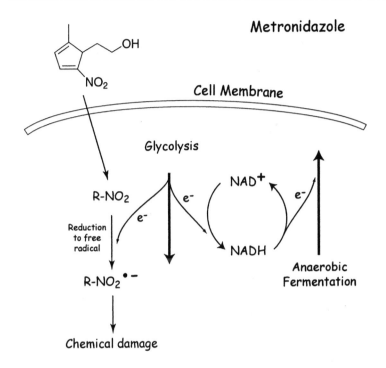

Metronidazole exerts two deleterious effects on anaerobic bacteria and protozoan parasites. First, upon reduction to a negatively charged highly reactive free radical, it chemically attacks diverse cellular materials and destroys their normal function. Because it is readily reduced and binds irreversibly to cell meterials, diffusion into the cell is nearly an irreversible process. Second, it consumes the reducing capacity of the cell, inhibiting the reduction of NAD+ to NADH which is needed for anaerobic fermentation.

Fig. 2.6.1

is a continuous gradient across the cell membrane from outside to inside, and biochemical damage accumulates. Second, this reaction competes for the reduction of NAD^+, and deprives the anaerobic cell of needed NADH.

Activity

Metronidazole is highly active against many Gram-negative anaer-obes, but it is inconsistently effective against Gram-positive anaerobes. It has important activity against *C. difficile, Helicobacter,* and several protozoa including trichomonas, ameba, and giardia.

Administration, Metabolism, and Elimination

Metronidazole is well absorbed and distributes well throughout all compartments including the cerebrospinal fluid and into abscesses.

Adverse Effects

Disulfiram-like reaction with alcohol. Glossitis and metallic taste. Neurotoxicity: siezures, encephalopathy, ataxia, and peripheral neuropathy.

Drug Interactions

Minor.

Mechanisms of Resistance

Resistance arises presumably as a result of the inactivation or loss of the enzyme that reduces the NO_2 group.

MUPIROCIN

Mupirocin is a bacterial product purified for topical use **(Fig. 2.6.2)**. It inhibits protein synthesis (by inhibiting the tRNA synthase for isoleucine), and its spectrum of action includes a variety of common Gram-positive skin pathogens, but not the normal flora of skin.

POLYPEPTIDES

Polypeptide antibiotics **(Fig. 2.6.2)** are ubiquitous in nature, and they even play a vital role in the host defense systems of humans. In most cases, their mechanisms of action are poorly defined, although they appear in general to alter membrane permeabilities. The action of gramicidin A is relatively well understood to be due to the formation of sodium ion channels. Systemic use is precluded by toxicity, but bacitracin, polymyxin B, and gramicidin have been widely employed for topical use. Being foreign polypeptides, these agents exhibit a high incidence of hypersensitivity reactions. This may be encountered in unexpected circumstances when small amounts of these com-pounds are included as preservatives in vaccines or other parenteral preparations.

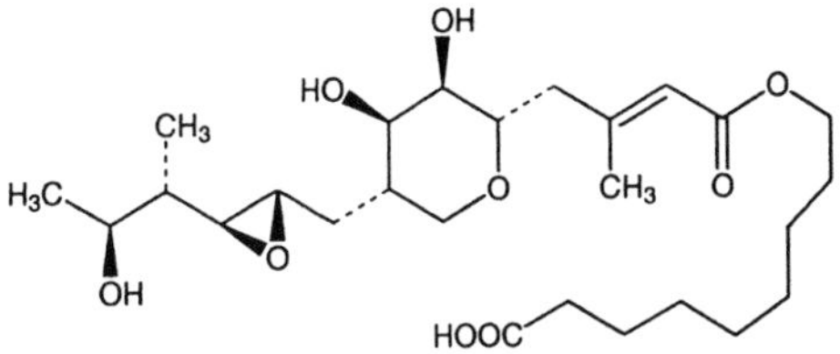

Mupirocin

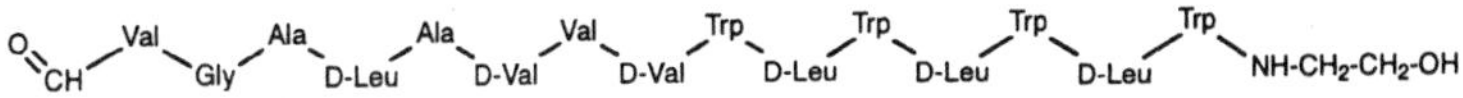

Gramicidin A

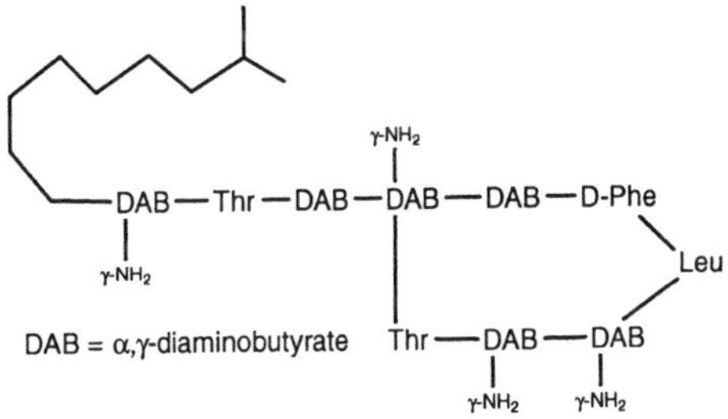

DAB = α,γ-diaminobutyrate

Polymyxin B

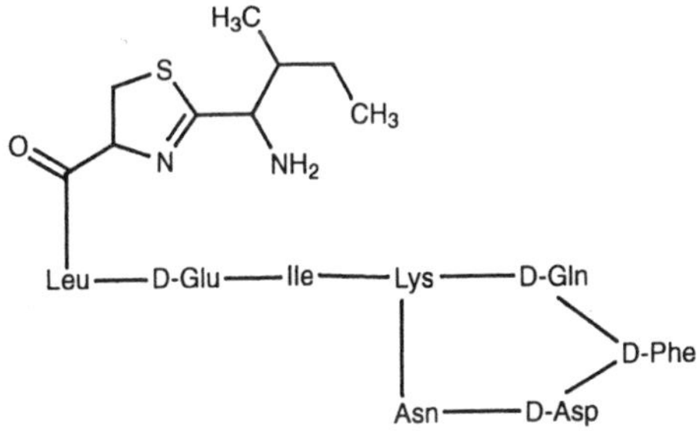

Bacitracin

Fig. 2.6.2

Table 2.7
Currently Marketed Antimycobacterial Agents

Generic name	Oral	IV	IM	Trade names
Aminosalicylic acid	X			Paser
Capreomycin		X	X	Capastat
Clofazimine	X			Lamprene
Ethambutol	X			Myambutol
Ethionamide	X			Trecator
Isoniazid	X		X	Rifater,[a] Nydrazid, Rifamate[a] Tubizid
Pyrazinamide	X			Rifater[a]
Rifabutin	X			Mycobutin
Rifampin	X	X		Rifamate,[a] Rifadin, Rimactane, Rifater
Rifapentine	X			Priftin

* Multicomponent product

O, oral; IV, intravenous; IM, intramuscular; T, topical, including preparations applied to skin, eyes, and ears

2.7 Antimycobacterial Agents (Table 2.7)

Drugs used for the treatment of tuberculosis have long been divided into first-line agents having relatively high efficacy and low toxicity, and second-line agents with either lower efficacy, higher toxicity, or both. Because resistance to any single agent arises spontaneously in a predictable fraction of organisms, but the likelihood that organisms will arise with simultaneous resistance to multiple agents is much lower, it is recommended that treatment always be initiated with multiple agents, particularly in cavitary lung disease where the numbers of organisms present may be large. For the same reason, drugs in a failing multidrug regimen are not replaced one at a time, but instead replaced with a new regimen incorporating at least two new drugs.

A distinction is made between the treatment of "active" or clinically apparent disease, and "latent" or subclinical disease. The latter is detected by a positive tuberculin skin test in someone who has not received effective antituberculous therapy. The treatment of subclinical infection is often referred to as "prophylaxis" or "prophylactic

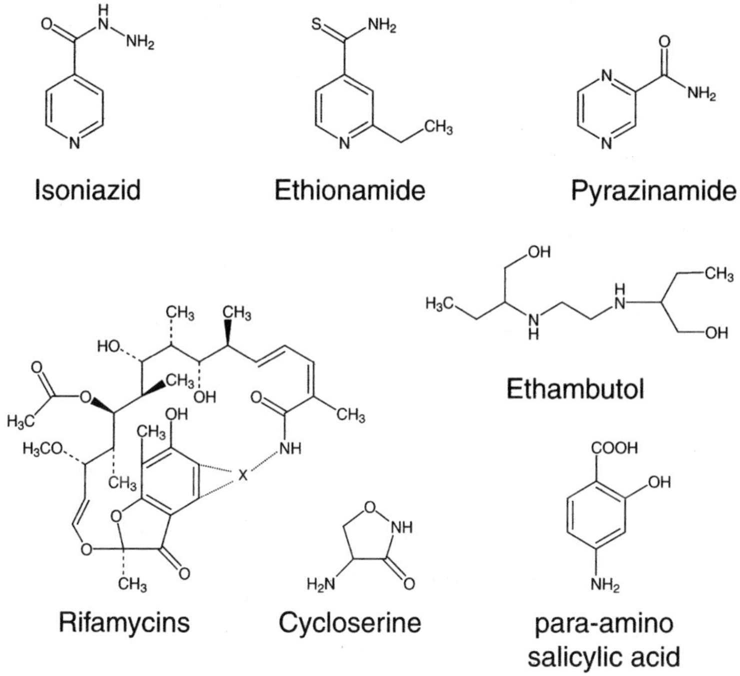

Isoniazid   Ethionamide   Pyrazinamide

Ethambutol

Rifamycins   Cycloserine   para-amino salicylic acid

Fig. 2.7

treatment" because it is aimed at preventing disease due to the reactivation of dormant tubercle bacilli later in life.

FIRST LINE AGENTS: ISONIAZID (INH)

Identity **(Fig. 2.7)**

Mechanism of Action

INH must be activated by a bacterial enzyme. The activated drug inhibits a key enzyme involved in mycolic acid synthesis

Activity

INH is an agent of choice for the treatment of latent infection and of active disease. The treatment of latent infection is generally prompted by a positive skin test with purified protein derivative (PPD) in the absence of evidence of active infection. Under these circumstances, the number of organisms present is believed to be sufficiently low to permit INH treatment of latent infection without problems arising due to INH resistance.

Administration, Metabolism, and Elimination

INH is acetylated by the liver and then eliminated into the urine. There is a bimodal distribution of genetic traits for rapid and slow rates of acetylation, but therapeutically adequate blood levels can be maintained with daily therapy even with rapid acetylators.

Adverse Effects

INH therapy is associated with a hepatotoxicity that may become life threatening, and whose incidence strongly correlates with age. It is also associated with peripheral neuropathy, whose incidence is strongly correlated with slow acetylation. Neuropathy is usually prevented by concomitant treatment with pyridoxine (vitamin B6).

Drug Interactions

There are numerous interactions between INH and other drugs, particularly in slow acetylators. Concomitant use of rifampin increases likelihood of hepatoxicity.

Resistance

Resistance arises via single step mutation in the activating enzyme. Mutations in the target enzyme (which confer cross-resistance to ethionamide) are less common.

FIRST LINE AGENTS: RIFAMYCINS

Identity **(Fig. 2.7)**

Rifamycins are complex bacterial products. Rifampin, rifapentine, and rifabutin (ansamycin) are semisynthetic derivatives.

Mechanism of Action

Rifamycins inhibit transcription (chain initiation by bacterial DNA-dependent RNA polymerase).

Activity

Rifamycins have broad antibacterial, antifungal, antiparasitic, and even antiviral activity. Rifampin is used as a single agent for prophylaxis against *N. meningitidis*, but it is not otherwise used as a single agent owing to rapid emergence of resistance. Its most important role is in multidrug programs for treating *M. tuberculosis*, and it may be used in combination with pyrazinamide for the treatment of latent infection (prophylactic treatment). Rifampin is also used occasionally to synergize with β-lactams against staphylococci and with amphotericin against candida. Rifabutin exhibits activity against some strains of *M. tuberculosis* that are resistant to rifampin, and it has better activity than rifampin against *M. avium* complex. Rifapentine has a longer half-life permitting less frequent dosing.

Administration, Metabolism, and Elimination

Rifamycins exhibit complex kinetics including autoinduction of metabolizing enzymes and interactions with isoniazid.

Adverse Effects

Rifamycins are associated with numerous adverse effects. All patients experience an orange-red coloration of the urine and tears that tends to permanently stain contact lenses. Many develop skin exanthems of varying severity and flu-like syndromes with long term treatment. Some develop hepatotoxicity and thrombocytopenia. Rifamycins increase the likelihood of hepatitis in patients treated with isoniazid.

Drug Interactions

Rifamycins induce hepatic microsomal enzymes leading to decreased effect of many drugs.

Resistance

Single step mutation in the target enzyme is common.

FIRST-LINE AGENTS: PYRAZINAMIDE (PZA)

PZA is a synthetic compound, similar to isoniazid and ethionamide in structure **(Fig. 2.7)**, and also similar in that it must be activated by cellular enzymes. These enzymes are peculiar to *M. tuberculosis*, so that PZA is not effective against other mycobacteria. Loss of its activating enzyme results in resistance. Although the target of the activated drug is not known, PZA is of proven value as a component of multidrug therapy for *M. tuberculosis* with a particular effectiveness against semidormant organisms. PZA can cause hyperuricemia. It also is associated with hepatotoxicity although it is not clear that this should be attributed to PZA because INH or rifampin are almost always given concomitantly, and these agents are hepatotoxic apart from PZA.

First-Line Agents: Ethambutol (EMB)

EMB is a simple synthetic compound **(Fig. 2.7)** that inhibits an enzyme involved in cell wall biosynthesis. It has proven value as a component of multidrug therapy for *M. tuberculosis,* but tends to cause optic neuritis with impairment of visual acuity and color vision at high doses.

First-Line Agents: Aminoglycosides

Streptomycin was the first aminoglycoside antibiotic to be used in humans (Section 2.3) and it shares most properties of other drugs in this class including their toxicities. Due to initial problems with vestibular toxicity when administered intravenously, it is now administered only via intramuscular injection. However, the tendency of streptomycin to cause this toxicity may not be greater than that of other aminoglycosides. It is highly active against *M. tuberculosis,* but is limited in its overall therapeutic efficacy because it is unable to reach intracellular organisms. Amikacin and kanamycin are also effective, but usually considered second line agents for historical reasons and relative cost.

Second-Line Agents: Quinolones

Quinolones (*see* Section 2.5) are being used with increasing frequency against *M. tuberculosis, M. avium* complex, and rapidly growing mycobacteria.

Second Line Agents: Paraaminosalicylic Acid (PAS)

PAS **(Fig. 2.7)** impairs folate synthesis but has weak antibacterial activity. Its limiting adverse effect is gastrointestinal disturbance.

Second-Line Agents: Cycloserine

Cycloserine **(Fig. 2.7)** is an analog of D-alanine that inhibits intracellular stages of cell wall biosynthesis (see discussion of glycopeptide antibiotics, above). It is associated with a high incidence of adverse effects, especially peripheral neuropathy and CNS/psychiatric disturbances.

Second-Line Agents: Ethionamide (ETH)

ETH **(Fig. 2.7)** is activated by a different enzyme than INH, but the activated drug inhibits the same enzymes responsible for mycolic acid synthesis as INH. Its limiting adverse effect is gastrointestinal disturbance.

OTHER SECOND-LINE AGENTS

Other compounds used against *M. tuberculosis* include capreomycin and viomycin (both cyclic polypeptides) and thiacetazone (a low-cost synthetic compound widely available in underdeveloped countries).

Clofazimine is a complex dye with an unknown mechanism of action, used primarily as part of combination therapy against *M. leprae.*

ß-lactams are active against the cell wall synthesizing enzymes of mycobacteria, but most mycobacteria resist this action by producing β-lactamases. β-Lactamase resistant cephalosporins are effective against rapidly growing mycobacteria, but not when the organisms are situated intracellularly (β-lactams cannot penetrate cell membranes.)

Macrolides are frequently active against various nontuberculous mycobacteria, and are especially useful in the prophylaxis and treatment of infections with *M. avium* complex.

Antifolate agents have activity against rapidly growing mycobacteria. The most important agent in this class is dapsone for its activity against *M. leprae.*

MULTIDRUG THERAPY AND MULTIDRUG RESISTANCE IN *M. TUBERCULOSIS*

Mutations that confer resistance to the drugs used for treating tuberculosis occur spontaneously with a rate of 10^{-3}–10^{-8}. Cavitary tuberculosis infections often involve more than 10^9 bacilli, and thus one can presume that organisms resistant to any one drug are present at the beginning of therapy. Therapy is usually initiated with multiple first-line agents because the probability of encountering spontaneous resistance to two or more drugs is the product of their individual probabilities. For example, one commonly used regimen consists of INH, rifampin, PZA, and EMB given for 2 m, followed by INH and rifampin for an additional 4 m. The choice of therapy in any particular individual, however, must consider local resistance patterns and any concomitant illness (such as HIV infection). When patient compliance with a prescribed treatment program is unreliable, threats to public health must be considered. Directly observed therapy (DOT) programs have been of proven value in such cases.

"Multidrug resistant" (MDR) tuberculosis is an infection with organisms resistant to INH and rifampin. Oftentimes, these organisms are resistant to other commonly used agents as well. MDR organisms tend to arise by serial selection of resistant mutants, as would occur when adding single agents to a failing treatment program, or when patient compliance is irregular.

2.8 Investigational Agents

New drugs are in development in each of the drug classes described above. In addition, several compounds belonging to entirely new drug classes are in development.

ADHESION BLOCKING AGENTS

There appears to be a potential for significant therapeutic value in blocking the mechanisms by which bacteria adhere to host tissues. Monoclonal antibodies directed against bacterial adhesins, and analogs of both bacterial adhesins and the adhesin targets of host tissues have demonstrated remarkable effectiveness in both animal and human models, including models of dental caries, candidiasis, various respiratory pathogens, and *Helicobacter* infections of the gut lumen.

DEFORMYLASE INHIBITORS

Bacteria synthesize proteins with a formyl (HCO–) group on the amino terminus that must be removed in most cases to form fully functional proteins. Inhibitors of deformylase such as actinonin are potently antibacterial, and are being developed as therapeutic agents.

DAPTOMYCIN

Daptomycin is a novel cyclic lipopeptide antibiotic that exerts its antibacterial effect at the bacterial cytoplasmic membrane and disrupts multiple aspects of membrane function, including peptidoglycan synthesis, lipoteichoic acid synthesis, and the bacterial membrane potential. Its mechanism of antimicrobial action is distinct from that of other antibiotics, including ß-lactams, aminoglycosides, glycopeptides, and macrolides. It is being developed for the treatment of Gram-positive infections such as staphylococci and enterococci.

EFFLUX PUMP INHIBITORS

Many instances of antimicrobial resistance are due to the active efflux of drugs from the bacterial cell by transmembrane energy-dependent pumps. Inhibitors of these pumps are being developed, with the intention of using them to suppress resistance to a co-administered antimicrobial agent.

EVERNINIMYCINS

Everninimycins (or everninomycins) belong to a class of oligosaccharide antibiotics with activity against Gram-positive bacteria. They bind to the 50S ribosomal subunit at a site distinct from currently available 50S-acting agents and inhibit protein synthesis. Unfortunately, one drug in this class—avilamycin—has been used extensively in Europe as an animal growth promoter and colonization of animals with bacteria resistant to both avilamycin and other everninimycins is prevalent. Possibly for this reason, the development of everninimycins for clinical use has been halted.

GLYCOPEPTIDES

Agents are under development that work by the same mechanism as vancomycin, but are effective against vancomycin resistant enterococci.

GLYCYLCYCLINES

Glycylcyclines are chemically related to tetracyclines, but will be designed to overcome tetracycline resistance among common respiratory pathogens.

POLYPEPTIDES

Polypeptides modeled after naturally occurring polypeptides known as "magainins" and "protegrins" are being developed for therapeutic use. Being foreign polypeptides, they are susceptible to digestion if given orally, and may be immunogenic if given parenterally. Current development is focused on topical agents and peptidomimetics that circumvent the problems inherent to ordinary polypeptides.

RAMOPLANIN

Ramoplanin is a complex natural product that binds to a membrane-anchored intermediate in cell wall biosynthesis and prevents its incorporation into peptidoglycan. Ramoplanin is highly effective against vancomycin-resistant enterococci, and is being developed for oral and topical administration to eliminate colonization by this organism in vulnerable populations.

2.9 Combination Antibacterial Therapy

There are four principal indications for using two or more antibiotics simultaneously to treat a patient with an infection.

1. Antibiotic combinations can prevent the emergence of resistance. This strategy is of proven value in the treatment of mycobacterial infections, and in the use of cotrimoxazole for various infections. However, this is not a universal advantage of combination therapy, and it is frequently cited to justify combination antibiotic therapy in situations where clinical data do not support this rationale.

2. In cases of polymicrobial infection combination therapy may be necessary because it is often not possible to choose a single antibiotic that is effective against all of the organisms that are present.

3. It is often the case that empiric treatment must be started while awaiting laboratory identification of the infecting organism. In these cases, it is often justifiable to begin therapy with a combination of antibiotics so that the possibility of treating with no effective agents is reduced.

4. Clinically useful synergism between antibiotics has been demonstrated in several clinical situations. However, not all synergy that is expected can be demonstrated in a laboratory, and not all that can be demonstrated is clinically useful.

Regardless of the indication, there are three disadvantages to combination antibiotic therapy in most clinical situations: it increases the number and likelihood of adverse effects or drug–drug interactions, there are additive costs, and there is the risk of unanticipated antagonism.

2.10 Choosing and Planning Antimicrobial Therapy

Historical information is needed before treatment planning to evaluate the likelihood of a bacterial infection, or the justification for prophylactic treatment. Once a need for treatment has been established, additional historical information is needed to ascertain the existence and nature of any hypersensitivity reactions, the most likely source of the infection (community, hospital, foreign), and host factors affecting antibiotic choice (coinfection with human immunodeficiency virus, immunosuppressive treatments, pregnancy, extreme age, recent prior antibiotic treatment). Finally, one adds local experience, epidemiological information, and formulary guidelines to this historical information and chooses among the subset of available antibiotics that have an appropriate spectrum of activity and the ability to penetrate to the site of the infection.

3 Antifungal Agents

(*See* **Table 3**)

3.1 Amphotericin

Amphotericin is member of a large family of compounds that also includes nystatin **(Fig. 3.1)**. Paradoxically, it is both a fungal product and a compound with potent antifungal activity. It is a chemically amphoteric molecule with large polar and nonpolar regions, but overall it is highly insoluble in water.

Mechanism of Action

Amphotericin binds to ergosterol in the cell wall of fungi and disrupts cell membrane permeability. It is moderately selective for ergosterol over cholesterol, although these targets are chemically similar, and imperfect selectivity of amphotericin for ergosterol undoubtedly contributes to the diversity and intensity of its adverse effects.

Activity

Amphotericin is active against nearly all pathological fungi. It also exhibits some activity against amoeba and *Leishmania*, although its mechanism of action against these organisms is unknown.

Administration, Metabolism, and Elimination

Due to insolubility in water, amphotericin is combined with deoxycholate and prepared as a fine colloidal suspension. The correct physical state of the suspension is critical for the efficient transfer of amphotericin from the suspension to the protein-bound state in plasma.

From: *Essentials of Antimicrobial Pharmacology*
By: P. H. Axelsen © Humana Press, Inc., Totowa, NJ

Table 3
Currently Marketed Antifungal Agents

Generic name	Oral	IV	IM	Top	Trade names
Amphotericin B	X	X		X	Fungizone, Amphotec, Abelcet, Amphocin, Ambisome
Butoconazole				X	Femstat
Ciclopirox				X	Penlac, Loprox
Clotrimazole	X			X	Fungoid,[a] Lotrisone, Lotrimin, Mycelex
Econazole				X	Spectazole
Fluconazole	X	X			Diflucan
Griseofulvin	X				Grisactin, Fulvicin, Fulvicin-U/F, Grifulvin, Gris, Gris-Peg
Itraconazole	X				Sporanox
Ketoconazole	X			X	Nizoral
Miconazole				X	Monistat-Derm, Monistat, Fungoid[a]
Nystatin	X			X	Myocidin, Mytrex, Mycolog, Mycostatin, Pedi, Mycogen, Nystop, Nilstat, Nystex
Oxiconazole				X	Oxistat
Potassium iodide	X			X	
Sulconazole				X	Exelderm
Terbinafine	X			X	Lamisil
Terconazole				X	Terazol
Tioconazole				X	Vagistat

[a]Multicomponent product

O, oral; IV, intravenous; IM, intramuscular; T, topical, including preparations applied to skin, eyes, and ears.

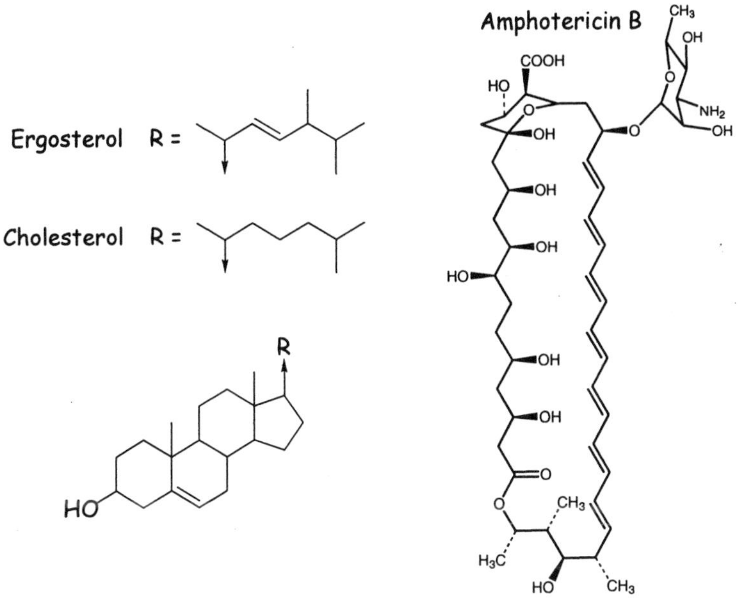

Fig. 3.1

To reduce toxicity, amphotericin has been combined with cholesterol, emulsified with lipids, or encapsulated in lipid vesicles (liposomes). Liposomal preparations enable much larger doses to be administered with minimal toxicity, but the kinetics and distribution of the drug are altered, and it is not yet clear that the larger doses lead to increased efficacy.

Because gastrointestinal absorption is minimal, oral administration is used only to treat fungal overgrowth in the gastrointestinal tract.

The penetration and elimination of amphotericin B into cerebro-spinal fluid and urine are limited, sometimes necessitating intrathecal and intravesicle administration for the treatment of brain and urinary tract infections.

A long tissue half-life (weeks to months) leads to courses of therapy that are measured in total dose, rather than duration of therapy. The rate at which amphotericin B can be administered is often limited to 0.5–1.5 mg/kg/d because higher daily doses tend to be excessively nephrotoxic.

Adverse Effects

Pyrexia and rigors are common during administration, most often necessitating premedication with antipyretics and analgesics. True hypersensitivity reactions, however, are uncommon.

Reversible nephrotoxicity is common, although it may require interruption of an administration schedule. The incidence and severity of nephrotoxicity are mitigated by salt and fluid loading prior to administration.

Mild anemia is common during therapy.

Drug Interactions

Amphotericin will precipitate upon mixing with saline prior to infusion. Caution must be exercised to avoid "piggybacking" an amphotericin suspension onto an intravenous infusion of saline.

Resistance

It is difficult to study and demonstrate amphotericin resistance for a variety of technical reasons. Some resistance appears to be due to reduced dependence on ergosterol, but these fungal strains may also be less pathogenic.

3.2 Flucytosine

Flucytosine (5-FC) is a structural analog of cytosine **(Fig. 3.2)**.

Mechanism of Action

5-FC is actively taken up by mechanisms that normally take up cytosine. It is converted to 5-fluorouracil (5-FU) in fungi, but not in mammalian cells. 5-FU inhibits thymidylate synthase and DNA synthesis. It is also incorporated into RNA and inhibits protein synthesis.

Activity

Chiefly used in combination with amphotericin against *Candida* and *Cryptococcus*.

Administration, Metabolism, and Elimination

Well absorbed orally, penetrates well into CSF, eliminated unchanged into the urine.

Adverse Effects

Bone marrow suppression. Gastrointestinal toxicity, potentially life threatening. Patients treated with 5-FC have been found to have

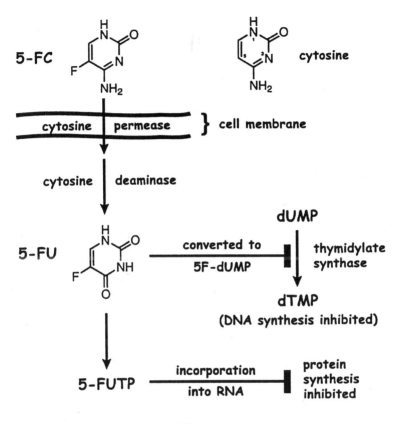

Fig. 3.2

varying amounts of 5-FU in their blood, in some cases as much as if the patient were being treated with 5-FU. The 5-FU may be produced from 5-FC by microbial flora in the gut, and may also be present in the 5-FC preparation as a result of spontaneous conversion during preparation, storage, and handling.

When 5-FC is administered with nephrotoxic agents (e.g., amphotericin), blood levels of 5-FC are often monitored to ensure that they are within a therapeutic but nontoxic range despite changes in renal function.

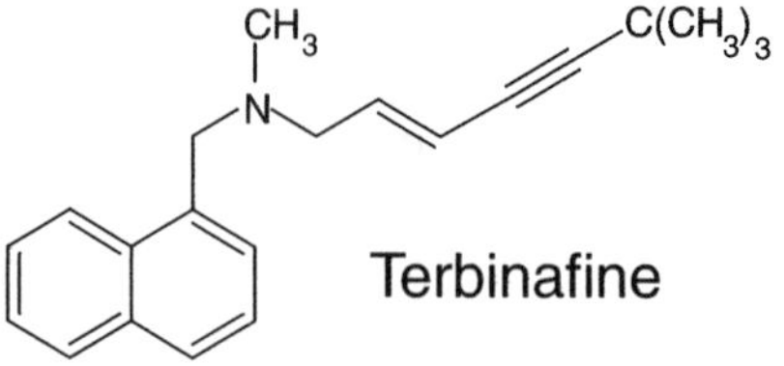

Fig. 3.3

Drug Interactions

5-FC acts synergistically to suppress the bone marrow when given with other bone marrow suppressive agents

Resistance

5-FC resistance arises commonly during therapy, due either to loss of cytosine uptake mechanism or loss of conversion enzyme.

3.3 Ergosterol Synthesis Inhibitors: Allylamines

Terbinafine **(Fig. 3.3)** inhibits an enzyme essential for the synthesis of ergosterol (a different enzyme than is inhibited by azoles). It is used topically for the treatment of dermatophytoses.

3.4 Ergosterol Synthesis Inhibitors: Azoles

Identity **(Fig. 3.4)**

There are many agents in this class, but most are too toxic for systemic use. The development of ketoconazole was significant for being the first orally administered agent active against deep mycoses.

Mechanism of Action

Azoles inhibit the cytochrome P-450-dependent synthesis of ergosterol (a different site than terbinafine).

Activity

There is significant variation in spectrum of activity among members of this class. Fluconazole is the most commonly used agent, with important roles in the treatment of *Candida*, *Cryptococcus*, and *Coccidioidomycosis* infections. Itraconazole has significantly broader activity, and is useful as a single agent in treating aspergillosis, histoplasmosis, blastomycosis, and onychomycosis. Ketoconazole

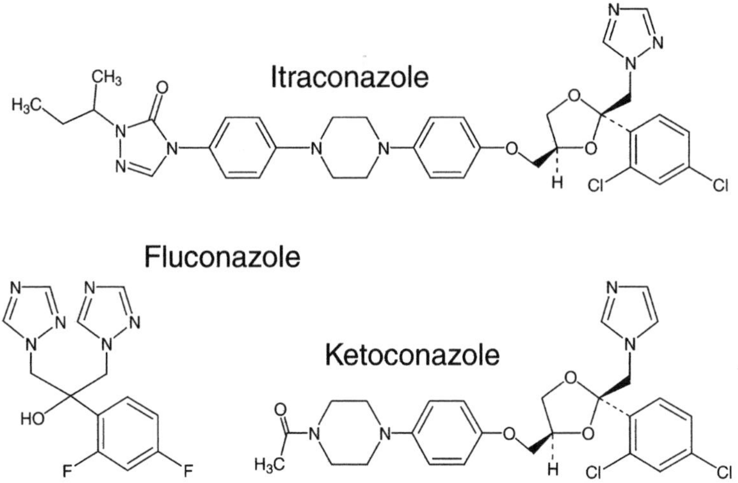

Fig. 3.4

was the first drug available in this class, and it represented a major breakthrough in the treatment of systemic mycoses. Although its role in oral therapy has been almost completely supplanted by itraconazole and fluconazole, it remains in common use as topical therapy.

Administration, Metabolism, and Elimination

Ketoconazole and itraconazole require stomach acid for absorption; fluconazole does not. Hepatic metabolism of ketoconazole becomes saturated at low levels, so that blood levels are not linearly related to dose. Itraconazole is converted in the liver to a compound with greater activity than the parent compound. Fluconazole is eliminated unchanged in the urine.

Adverse Effects

Ketoconazole causes gastrointestinal disturbances and disrupts steroid endocrine systems. Itraconazole has fewer adverse effects, and those of fluconazole are relatively mild.

Drug Interactions

Azole drugs participate in numerous significant drug–drug interactions because their primary mechanism of action is to inhibit a hepatic

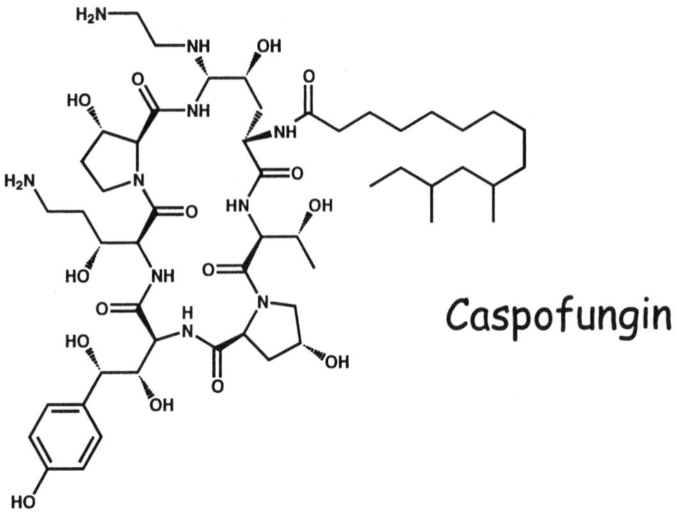

Fig. 3.5

cytochrome P-450 system. This enzyme system is involved in the metabolism of many other drugs, e.g., benzodiazepines, HMG-CoA reductase inhibitors, immunosuppresants, hypoglycemic agents, and HIV protease inhibitors.

Resistance

There are multiple incompletely defined mechanisms of resistance.

3.5 Caspofungin

Caspofungin is the first drug in a new class of drugs called echinocandins that inhibit the synthesis of β(1-3)-D-glucan, an essential component of the fungal cell wall. It is a complex semisynthetic lipopeptide derived from bacteria (Fig 3.5) with activity against several species of *Aspergillus*.

3.6 Griseofulvin

Griseofulvin binds to microtubules and inhibits mitosis. It is useful against against dermatophytic fungi because it is concentrated in keratinocytes, although it has numerous side effects and drug–drug interactions.

4 Antiparasitic Agents

See **Table 4.1**.

The most important distinction of pharmacological significance to the treatment of parasitic infections is whether the infecting organism is a unicellular protozoan or a multicellular helminth **(Table 4.2)**. Most antiparasitic agents have a relatively broad spectrum of activity within one of these groups, but virtually no crossover activity in the other group. Mechanisms of action for many antiparasitic agents are not known. Some of the most effective treatments for parasitic infections are not commonly used in the United States, and are therefore either not available or must be obtained through special channels.

4.1. Antiprotozoan Agents

4.1.1 Metronidazole

Metronidazole **(Fig. 2.1.6)** is active against most luminal protozoa, but is especially useful for its ability to treat extraluminal infections such as amebic liver abscess. Protozoa are susceptible to the action of metronidazole because they share the same activating enzyme as anaerobic bacteria. Protozoa, however, are much less likely to have acquired resistance than bacteria. This is presumably because protozoa are diploid and, therefore single mutations cannot stop metronidazole activation. Metronidazole is not active against amebic cysts. Related drugs are available outside the United States. See discussion of the antibacterial activity of metronidazole, section 2.1.6.

From: *Essentials of Antimicrobial Pharmacology*
By: P. H. Axelsen © Humana Press, Inc., Totowa, NJ

31654992924114496073359829063562910191

Table 4.1
Currently Marketed Antiparasitic Agents

Generic name	Oral	IV	IM	I	Trade names
Albendazole	X				Albenza
Atovaquone	X				Mepron
Chloroquine	X		X		Aralen
Furazolidone	X				Furoxone
Halofantrine	X				Halfan
Hydroxychloroquine	X				Plaquenil
Iodoquinol	X				Yodoxin
Ivermectin	X				Stromectol, Mectizan
Mebendazole	X				Vermox
Mefloquine	X				Lariam
Paromomycin	X				Humatin
Pentamidine		X	X	X	Pentacarinat, Pentam, Nebupent
Praziquantel	X				Biltricide
Pyrimethamine	X				Daraprim,[a] Fansidar[a]
Quinidine	X				Quinaglute, Quinidex, QuinTabs, QuinaDure
Quinine	X				
Thiabendazole	X				Mintezol

[a]Multicomponent product
O, oral; IV, intravenous; IM, intramuscular, I, inhaled

4.1.2 Emetine / Dehydroemetine (Fig 4.1.2)

A relatively toxic treatment for extraintestinal amebic infection, e.g. amebic abscess. Derived from ipecac, with which it shares adverse effects (induction of emesis, hence its name). These drugs work by inhibiting protein synthesis in ameba trophozoites, but they have no effect on amebic cysts.

4.1.3 Iodoquinol (Fig. 4.1.3)

Orally administered and poorly absorbed agent used to eradicate protozoan cysts. Usually administered as follow-up treatment for extraintestinal amebic infections.

4.1.4 Diloxanide Furoate (Fig. 4.1.2)

Low-cost treatment for asymptomatic intestinal amebic infections and cyst eradication.

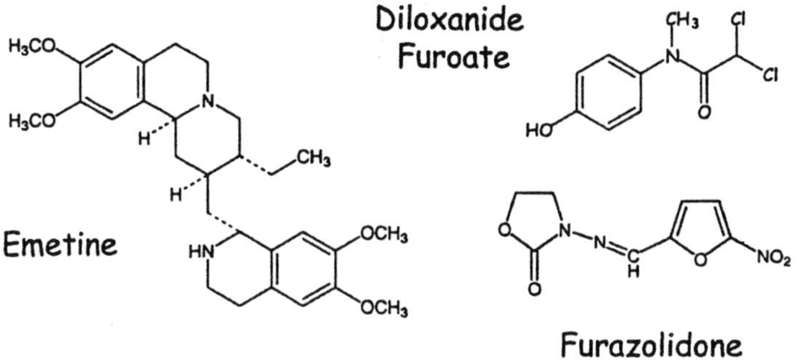

Fig. 4.1.2

4.1.5 Paromomycin

An aminoglycoside that may be orally administered for the treatment of asymptomatic intestinal amebic infections because it is poorly absorbed. Reportedly effective in some cases against cryptosporidia.

4.1.6 Quinacrine

Identity (**Fig. 4.1.3**)

Mechanism of Action

Quinacrine intercalates into DNA and inhibits DNA polymerase. However, it is unclear whether these properties are related to its antiparasitic effect.

Activity

Lowest cost and most effective treatment for giardiasis. Historically, it has also been used against malaria and tapeworms.

Administration, Metabolism, and Elimination

Well absorbed, binds tightly to various tissues resulting in prolonged elimination over months.

Adverse Effects

Quinacrine typically causes a yellow discoloration of the skin. Gastrointestinal and central nervous system (CNS) disturbances are common, including toxic psychosis, and an antabuse reaction with ethanol.

Table 4.2
Classification of Human Parasites

Protozoa	Luminal		*Entamoeba histolytica* *Giardia lamblia* *Trichomonas vaginalis* *Blastocystis* *Balantidium coli*
	Tissue	Apicomplexa	*Plasmodium* spp. *Babesia bigemina* *Toxoplasma gondii* *Cryptosporidium parvum* *Isospora belli*
		Pneumocystis carinii	
		Trypanosomes	*Leishmania* American (Chagas disease) African (African sleeping sickness)
Helminths	Nematodes (roundworms)	Luminal	*Ascaris* spp. (roundworm) *Trichuris* spp. (whipworm) *Enterobius vermicularis* (pinworm)
		Tissue	*Trichinella spiralis* (trichinosis) *Strongyloides stercoralis* (strongyloidiasis) *Toxocara canis* (visceral larva migrans) *Ancylostoma* spp. (cutaneous larva migrans) *Necator americanus* (hookworm) *Angiostrongylus catonensis* *Brugia malayi* (filariasis) *Wuchereria bancrofti* (filariasis) *Loa loa* (African eye worm) *Onchocerca volvulus* (onchocerciasis, African river blindness) *Dracunculus* (Guinea worm)

| Helminths | Cestodes (flatworms) | Echinococcus granulosis
Echinococcus multilocularis
Taenia spp. (cysticercosis)
Diphyllobothrium latum (sparganosis)
Fasciola hepatica |
| | Trematodes (flukes) | Clonorchis sinensis
Shistosoma spp.
Paragonimus westermani |

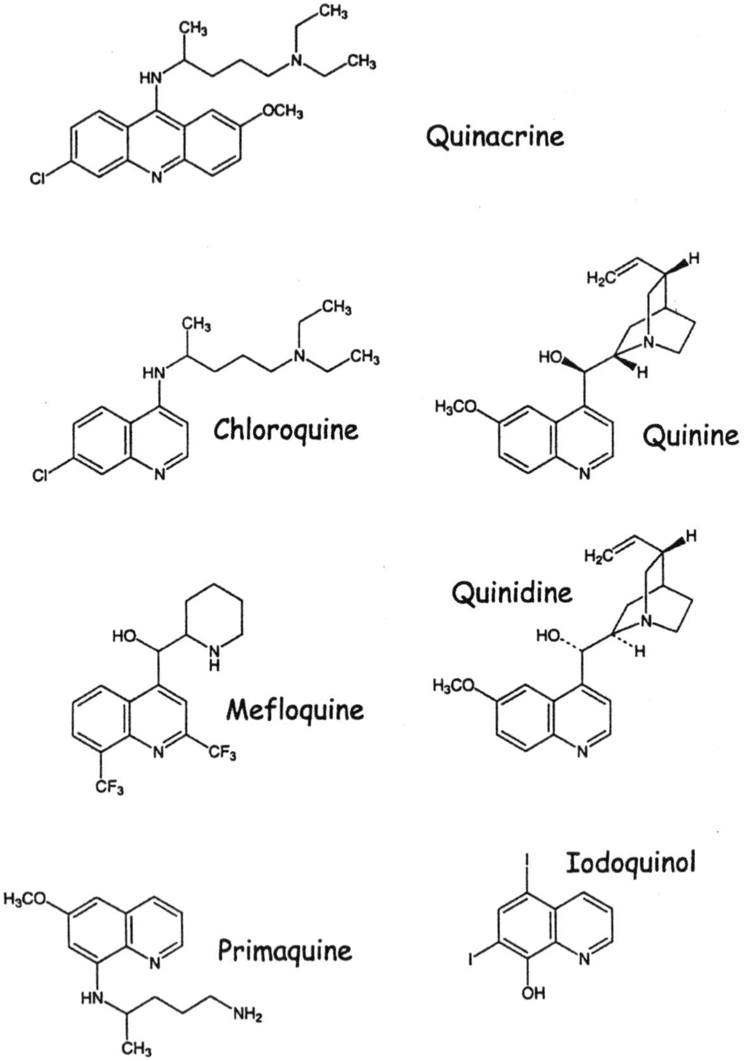

Quinacrine

Chloroquine

Quinine

Mefloquine

Quinidine

Primaquine

Iodoquinol

Fig. 4.1.3

Drug Interactions

Strongly inhibits metabolism of primaquine

4.1.7 Quinolines

Identity **(Fig. 4.1.3)**

Mechanism of Action

These drugs are concentrated in erythrocytes parasitized with malaria, where they bind with high affinity to hemoglobin degradation products in the parasite's digestive vesicles. Binding appears to interfere with normal processing of digestive vesicles by the parasite.

Activity

Chloroquine used for prophylaxis and treatment of *P. vivax*, *P. ovale*, and *P. malaria*. Mefloquine used for prophylaxis and treatment of all forms of malaria including *P. falciparum* strains resistant to chloroquine and quinine. Quinine and quinidine used primarily for the treatment of chloroquine-resistant *P. falciparum*.

Administration, Metabolism, and Elimination

Chloroquine and mefloquine have long serum half-lives that allow once-per-week dosing for prophylaxis.

Adverse Effects

Mefloquine is associated with high incidence of sinus bradycardia, although this has no apparent long-term sequelae. The mechanism is unknown. Serious neuropsychiatric disturbances occur in patients taking treatment courses, but are relatively rare in patients on prophylactic doses.

A well known array of adverse effects due to quinine is known as "cinchonism" and consists of tinnitus, hearing loss, visual symptoms, headache, and gastrointestinal disturbances. Quinine also has a curare-like effect on skeletal muscle that is useful in the treatment of nocturnal leg cramps.

Resistance

Active efflux renders many strains of *P. falciparum* chloroquine resistant. Some evidence suggests that calcium channel blockers (e.g., verapamil) may inhibit this efflux and negate chloroquine resistance. Resistance to quinine, quinidine, and mefloquine is also found in regions of Africa and Southeast Asia.

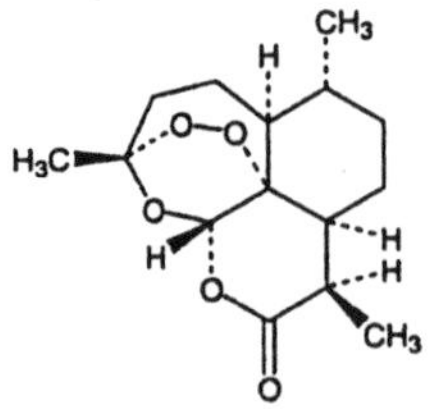

Artemisinine 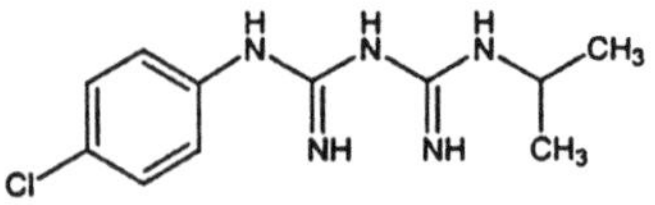   **Proguanil**

Fig. 4.1.11

4.1.8 Primaquine

Primaquine (**Fig. 4.1.3**) is believed to interfere with electron transport or nucleic acid synthesis. It is the only drug known to be effective at eliminating the hepatic (exoerythrocytic) stages of *P. vivax* and *P. ovale*. It is also effective against the gametocyte stages of all four *Plasmodium* species. Primaquine is primarily used to provide "radical" cure of latent infection after chloroquine treatment or prophylaxis. Daily oral administration for 14 d is necessary to eradicate exoerythrocytic parasites. Persons with G6PD deficiency are at risk of hemolysis (5–10% incidence in Chinese and African males).

4.1.9 Furazolidone (Fig. 4.1.2)

Useful for treating giardiasis in small children because it is available in an orally-administered liquid form. Mechanism of action likely related to that of metronidazole (note presence of "nitro" group). Like metronidazole, causes an disulfiram-like reaction with alcohol.

4.1.10 Tetracycline and Doxycycline

Tetracyclines are effective for the prophylaxis and treatment of *P. falciparum* strains resistant to chloroquine and quinine. Photosensitivity is a serious potential problem because intense sun exposure frequently accompanies the risk of malaria exposure.

4.1.11 Artemisinin (Fig. 4.1.11)

A traditional Chinese natural product also known as Qinghaosu, with activity against *P. falciparum* strains resistant to chloroquine and quinine. Its mechanism of action is unknown, but is believed to alter the integrity of Plasmodia membranes.

4.1.12 Antifolate Agents

Proguanil (Fig. 4.1.11) was the first antifolate agent used for malaria prophylaxis and treatment. It is concentrated in erythrocytes and converted to an active metabolite that inhibits dihydrofolate reductase. It is not adequate for prophylaxis as a single agent, however, because *P. vivax* can develop resistance. The combination of proguanil and atovaquone (section 4.1.14) has recently been approved for the prevention and treatment of *P. falciparum* infections.

Trimethoprim/sulfamethoxazole (cotrimoxazole) is effective for prophylaxis and treatment of *Pneumocystis* infections, and commonly used in patients with HIV infection and low CD4 cell counts.

Pyrimethamine selectively inhibits dihydrofolate reductase in *Plasmodia, Pneumocystis,* and *Toxoplasma.* Combined with sulfadoxime (Fansidar) it is effective for effective for prophylaxis and treatment of chloroquine-resistant malaria, although the risk of death due to hypersensitivity reactions caused by the sulfonamide component may be as high as the risk of death due to malaria. Combined with dapsone (Maloprim) it is used for the prophylaxis of malaria and *Pneumocystis.*

4.1.13 Pentamidine

Pentamidine (Fig. 4.1.13) is used almost exclusively against *Pneumocystis* in patients intolerant of cotrimoxazole, but it is also active against some trypanosomes and Leishmania. Its mechanism of action is unclear, but it appears to induce multifaceted biochemical dysfunction. Inhaled aerosolized pentamidine is minimally absorbed into the systemic circulation. When administered intravenously or intramuscularly, it is tightly bound to tissues and elimination is prolonged over many days. Aside from a tendency to provoke bronchospasm, inhaled pentamidine aerosol is well tolerated. Intravenous administration is associated with severe hypoglycemia, renal failure, and a variety of hematologic, biochemical, and CNS disturbances.

4.1.14 Atovaquone

Atovaquone (Fig. 4.1.13) is a synthetic compound that is active against malaria, pneumocystis, and toxoplasma. In combination with

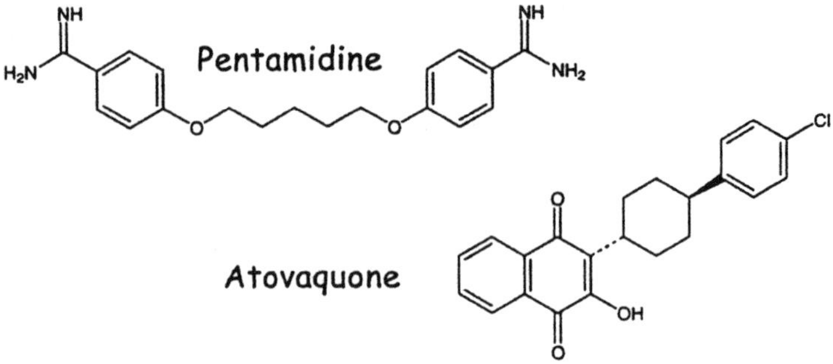

Fig. 4.1.13

azithromycin, atovaquone has recently been recommended as first-line treatment for babesiosis. In combination with proguanil (Section 4.1.12), it may be used for the prevention and treatment of *P. falciparum* infections. It appears to work by interfering with electron transport in parasite mitochondria. Although it is poorly absorbed from the gastrointestinal tract, enough is absorbed for it to be effective for the prophylaxis of pneumocystis pneumonia in persons with advanced HIV infection.

4.1.15 Agents Effective Against Trypanosomes

Drugs of choice for the treatment of trypanosomiasis are not routinely available in the United States.

SURAMIN

Suramin is used to treat early stages of African sleeping sickness (*Trypanosoma brucei* spp) and adult *Onchocerca*. It does not penetrate the CNS, therefore is not useful against advanced sleeping sickness. It causes numerous and serious adverse effects.

MELARSOPROL

A trivalent arsenic-containing compound that is effective for the treatment of advanced African sleeping sickness because it penetrates the CNS. It causes numerous and serious adverse effects.

EFLORNITHINE

A potent enzyme-activated inhibitor of ornithine decarboxylase that is active against early and CNS stages of African sleeping sickness, and has relatively mild adverse effects. It is also useful in cases of *Pneumocystis* refractory to other treatments. A topical form of eflornithine is used in the U.S. for the treatment of hirsuitism.

NIFURTIMOX / BENZNIDAZOLE

Nitrofuran and nitroimidazole derivatives with useful but inconsistent activity against Chagas' disease (*Trypanosoma cruzi*), and a high incidence of serious side effects. Their mechanism of action most likely involves the formation of highly reactive free radicals (see metronidazole).

ANTIMONY

Several agents containing pentavalent antimony are active against *Leishmania* spp. and are generally well tolerated.

4.2 Antihelminthic Agents

4.2.1 Luminal Roundworms

MEBENDAZOLE, ALBENDAZOLE (FIG. 4.2.1)

These drugs inhibit glucose uptake and microtubule assembly. They are broadly active against ascaris, hookworms, whipworms, and pinworms. Albendazole is recommended for the treatment of inoperable echinococcus. Low bioavailability results in minimal systemic side effects, but makes it difficult to use against systemic nematodes

THIABENDAZOLE (FIG. 4.2.1)

This drug probably inhibits microtubule assembly, and is broadly useful against systemic nematodes including *Strongyloides*, cutaneous and visceral larva migrans, and *Trichinella*. As a consequence of being better absorbed than mebendazole, it also has a higher incidence of gastrointestinal, CNS, biochemical and hematologic side effects.

PYRANTEL (FIG. 4.2.2)

Pyrantel is effective against ascaris, hookworms, and pinworms, but not whipworms. It acts by depolarizing neuromuscular junctions and inhibiting acetylcholinesterases, resulting in spastic paralysis. For this reason, it antagonizes the action of piperazine.

PIPERAZINE (FIG. 4.2.2)

Piperazine is effective against ascaris and pinworms. It acts by hyperpolarizing muscle membranes and causing flaccid paralysis. This action does not kill worms, and is antagonized by pyrantel.

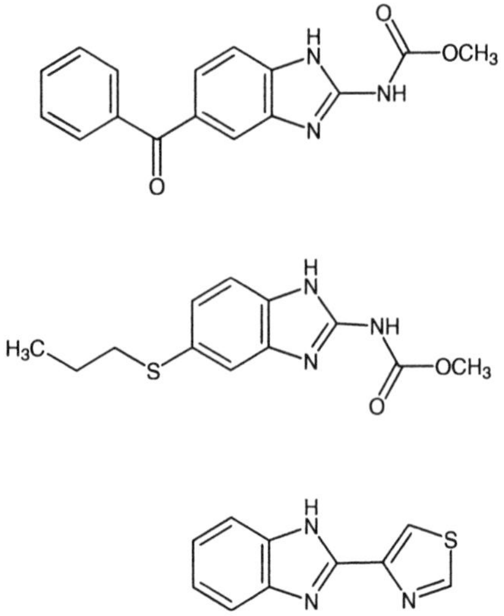

Mebendazole

Albendazole

Thiabendazole

Fig. 4.2.1

4.2.2 Systemic Roundworms

DIETHYLCARBAMAZINE

Diethylcarbamazine **(Fig. 4.2.2)** is a derivative of piperazine that hyperpolarizes muscle membranes resulting in flaccid paralysis, probably due to its piperazine moiety. It also appears to render parasite membranes more susceptible to host defense mechanisms. It is rapidly active against microfilarial worms including *Loa loa* and *Onchocerca*, but does not kill adult *Onchocerca* (must use Suramin). It is used presumptively in cases of tropical eosinophilia to treat filariasis. Rapid action can result in an intense inflammatory reaction due to the release of parasitic antigens (the Mazotti reaction). Often administered with steroids to reduce the reaction intensity, particularly in cases of ocular infection.

IVERMECTIN (FIG. 4.2.2)

Ivermectin is an agonist of several types of ligand-gated chloride ion channel receptors. The target in parasitic helminths is a glutamate

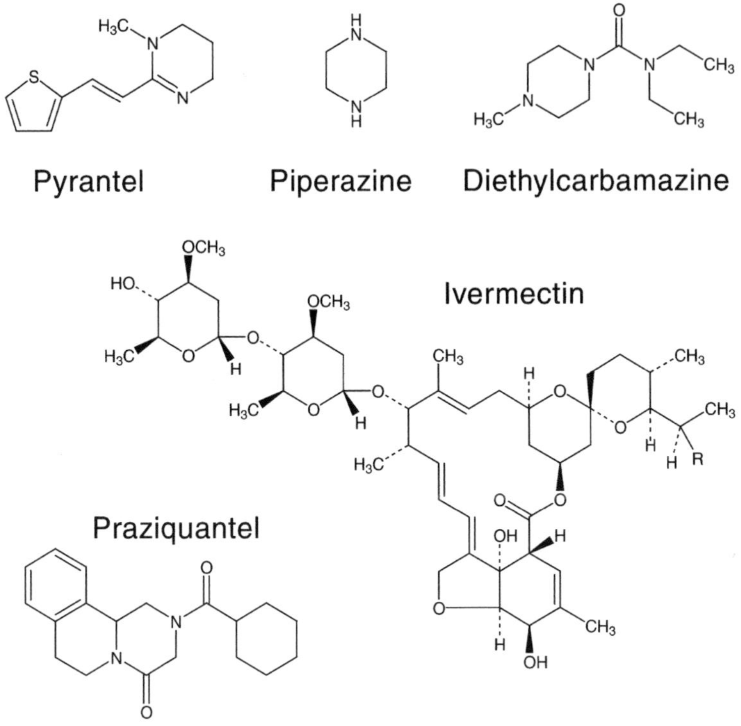

Pyrantel   Piperazine   Diethylcarbamazine

Ivermectin

Praziquantel

Fig. 4.2.2

receptor which, when stimulated to conduct chloride ions, blocks synaptic transmission. It is used chiefly against *Onchocerca* and microfilaria. It inhibits egg production, but does not kill parasites. Compared to diethylcarbamazine, it acts more slowly, is much less likely to elicit a strong inflammatory reaction, and is overall better tolerated.

4.2.3 Tapeworms / Flukes

PRAZIQUANTEL (FIG. 4.2.2)

Praziquantel has broad activity against shistosomes, larval and adult tapeworms, and flukes. It is especially useful in treating cysticercosis and acts by increasing membrane permeability to calcium, resulting in tetanic contractures. It is well tolerated, although parasite antigens may induce intense inflammatory responses.

NICLOSAMIDE

Niclosamide is active against adult tapeworms. It uncouples oxidative phosphorylation, resulting in death and disintegration of the worm. It does not kill larval forms, so autoreinfection is possible. To prevent reinfection, one may purge the gastrointestinal tract after treatment, or use praziquantel instead. The drug is well tolerated owing to minimal systemic absorption.

OXAMNIQUINE

Used to treat *Shistosoma mansoni*; less expensive than praziquantel.

5 Antiviral Agents

(*See* **Table 5**)

Viral replication depends on many of the same cellular processes that operate in normal uninfected cells. As a consequence, relatively few essential processes are unique to virally infected cells, and it is difficult to identify, target, and inactivate these processes in infected cells without harming uninfected host cells. It is also difficult to develop broad-spectrum agents because the targeted process is often specific to one type of virus.

5.1 Antiherpesvirus Agents

All available antiherpesvirus agents target the virally encoded DNA polymerases that replicate the double-stranded DNA genomes of these viruses. Viral DNA polymerases operate in the same manner as cellular DNA polymerases, (i.e., they join the 5'-OH group of the base being added to the 3'-OH group of a 2'-deoxyribose sugar in the polymerized strand of DNA).

5.1.1 Purine Analogs

Identity (**Fig. 5.1.1.1**)

The purine analogs used against herpesviruses all lack the cyclic deoxyribose sugar of 2'-deoxyguanosine. The first drug in this class was given the prefix "acyclo" for this reason.

Mechanism of Action (**Fig. 5.1.1.2**)

Acyclovir is taken up by cells and monophosphorylated by a herpesvirus, (HSV)-encoded thymidine kinase. Cellular enzymes

From: *Essentials of Antimicrobial Pharmacology*
By: P. H. Axelsen © Humana Press, Inc., Totowa, NJ

Table 5
Currently Marketed Antiviral Agents

Generic name	Chief use	O	IV	IM	SQ	T	Trade names
Abacavir	HIV	X					Ziagen
Acyclovir	HSV	X	X			X	Zovirax
Amantadine	Influenza A	X					Symmetrel
Amprenavir	HIV	X					Agenerase
Cidofovir	CMV		X				Vistide
Delavirdine	HIV	X					Rescriptor
Didanosine	HIV	X					Videx
Efavirenz	HIV	X					Sustiva
Famciclovir	HSV	X					Famvir
Foscarnet	HSV, CMV		X				Foscavir
Ganciclovir	CMV	X	X				Cytovene
Indinavir	HIV	X					Crixivan
Lamivudine	HIV	X					Epivir, Combivir[a]
Lopinavir	HIV	X					Kaletra[a]
Nelfinavir	HIV	X					Viracept
Nevirapine	HIV	X					Viramune
Oseltamivir	Influenza A,B	X					Tamiflu
Penciclovir	HSV					X	Denavir
Ribavirin	RSV	X				X	Virazole, Rebetol
Rimantadine	Influenza A	X				X	Flumadine
Ritonavir	HIV	X					Norvir, Kaletra[a]
Saquinavir	HIV	X					Invirase, Fortovase
Stavudine	HIV	X					Zerit
Trifluridine	HSV					X	Viroptic
Valacyclovir	HSV	X					Valtrex
Valganciclovir	CMV	X					Valcyte
Vidarabine	HSV					X	Vira-A
Zalcitabine	HIV	X					Hivid
Zanamivir	Influenza A,B					X	Relenza
Zidovudine	HIV	X	X				Combivir,[a] Retrovir

[a]In combination with ritonavir

HIV, human immunodeficiency virus; HBV, hepatitis B virus; HCV, hepatitis C virus; HSV, herpes simplex virus; HPV, human papilloma virus; VZV, Varicella-zoster virus; CMV, cytomegalovirus; EBV, Epstein-Barr virus

O, oral; IV, intravenous; IM, intramuscular; SQ, subcutaneous; T, topical, including inhaled preparations and those applied to skin, eyes, and ears

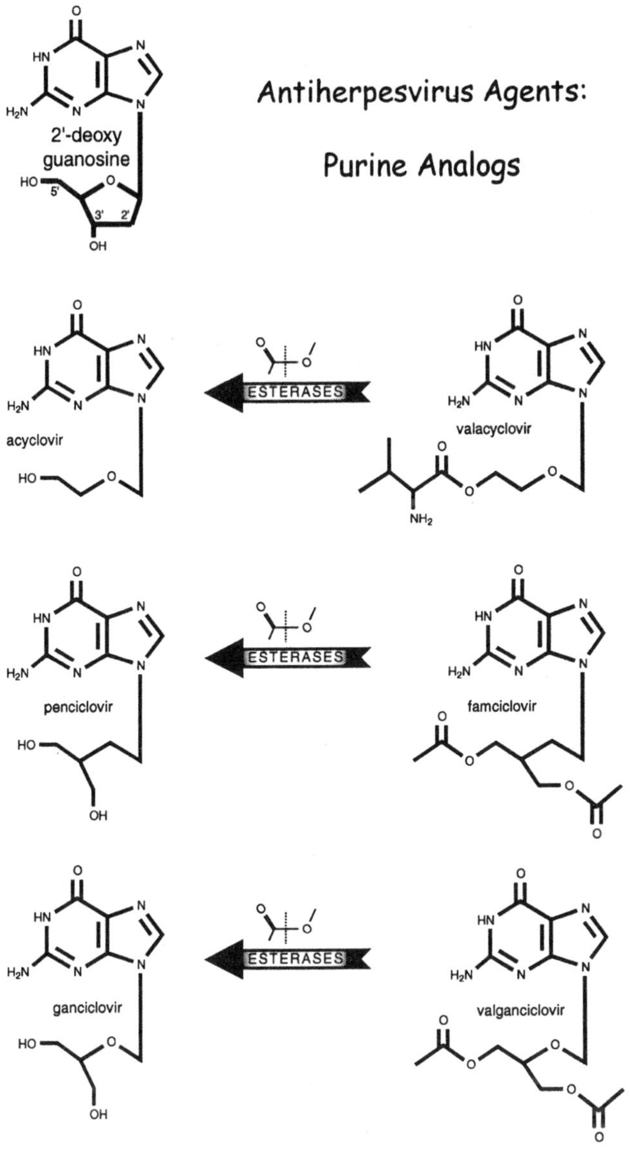

Antiherpesvirus Agents:

Purine Analogs

2'-deoxy
guanosine

acyclovir

ESTERASES

valacyclovir

penciclovir

ESTERASES

famciclovir

ganciclovir

ESTERASES

valganciclovir

Fig. 5.1.1.1

Purines and Purine Analogs in Cells Infected with Herpesviruses

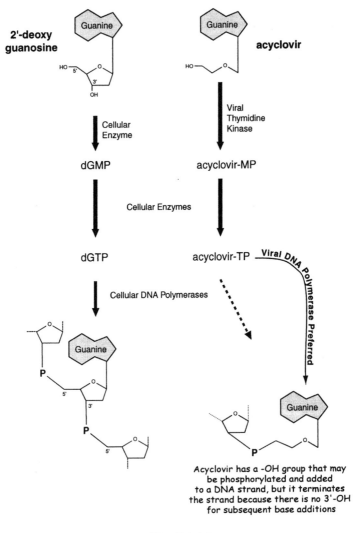

Acyclovir has a -OH group that may be phosphorylated and added to a DNA strand, but it terminates the strand because there is no 3'-OH for subsequent base additions

Fig. 5.1.1.2

then convert it to the triphosphate form. Acyclovir triphosphate competitively inhibits viral DNA polymerase. In addition, it can be added by DNA polymerase to the 3'-OH of a strand of DNA, but it has no corresponding 3'-OH to which additional nucleotides may be added. This terminates the DNA strand and permanently inactivates the enzyme.

Acyclovir acts selectively against virally infected cells because (1) only virally infected cells have the thymidine kinase required to monophosphorylate the drug, and (2) the drug preferentially binds to the virally encoded DNA polymerase.

Ganciclovir and penciclovir are also competitive inhibitors of DNA polymerase, but they have analogs of 3'-OH, and will permit chain extension. Ganciclovir is monophosphorylated by a phosphotransferase encoded by cytomegalovirus, (CMV). This enzyme is not as effective on acyclovir and thus, ganciclovir is more effective than acyclovir against CMV-infected cells.

Activity

Acyclovir is used primarily for HSV infections, and occasionally for varicella–zoster virus, (VZV) infections. Ganciclovir is used almost exclusively for CMV infections. The activity of penciclovir more closely resembles that of acyclovir, despite its closer chemical resemblance to ganciclovir. None of these agents exhibit useful activity against Epstein–Barr virus.

Administration, Metabolism, and Elimination

Acyclovir and ganciclovir are poorly absorbed from the gastrointestinal tract, but therapeutically effective levels can nonetheless be achieved by this route. Penciclovir is not absorbed to any useful degree and is used only topically. Valacyclovir is well absorbed from the gastrointestinal tract and readily converted to acyclovir by esterases in the gut and liver. It yields much higher plasma levels of acyclovir than does oral administration of acyclovir. Famciclovir and valganciclovir are well absorbed from the gastrointestinal tract and acted upon by esterases to yield therapeutically useful levels of penciclovir and ganciclovir.

All drugs in this class are eliminated by the kidneys and have relatively short plasma half-lives, 2–3 h. However, their intracellular half-lives correlate better to their activity. The intracellular half-life of acyclovir is shorter than its plasma half-life, but its effects persist because it permanently inactivates DNA polymerase. The intracellular half-lives of ganciclovir (~12 h) and penciclovir (up to 20 h) are much longer.

Adverse Effects

Acyclovir and penciclovir are associated with gastrointestinal and CNS disturbances. Ganciclovir is known to cause bone marrow depression, or to aggravate marrow suppression caused by other drugs.

Drug Interactions

No consistent interactions of major clinical importance.

Resistance

The most common form of resistance is due to the absence of viral thymidine kinase activity. Less commonly, the viral thymidine kinase loses an ability to phosphorylate acyclovir, but retains an ability to phosphorylate thymidine. In some cases, mutations of viral DNA polymerase have caused resistance.

5.1.2 Pyrimidine Analogs (Fig. 5.1.2)

CIDOFAVIR

Identity

A nucleoside phosphonate analog of cytosine.

Mechanism

Cidofavir is converted by host cell enzymes to a diphosphoryl derivative that selectively inhibits the DNA polymerase of CMV.

Activity

Owing to its high toxicity, usage is limited to the treatment of CMV retinitis in persons with advanced HIV infection.

Administration, Metabolism, and Elimination

Intravenous administration must be preceded by the oral administration of probenecid. This inhibits the secretion of cidofavir into the proximal renal tubules and thereby protects against nephrotoxicity.

Adverse Effects

Severe nephrotoxicity, neutropenia.

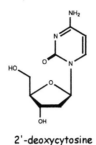

2'-deoxycytosine

Antiherpesvirus Agents:

Pyrimidine Analogs

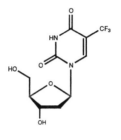

Trifluridine   Idoxuridine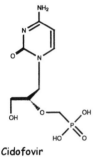

Cidofovir

Fig. 5.1.2

Drug Interactions

Probenecid alters the pharmacokinetics of many other agents. Concomitant administration of other nephrotoxic agents is contraindicated.

Resistance

There is some cross resistance with ganciclovir, but cross-resistance with foscarnet is uncommon.

IDOXURIDINE

Idoxuridine is a pyrimidine analog that is phosphorylated by viral thymidine kinase and competitively inhibits DNA polymerase. Poor selectivity for virally infected cells limits its application to the topical treatment of corneal infections with HSV. Low or absent thymidine kinase is associated with viral resistance.

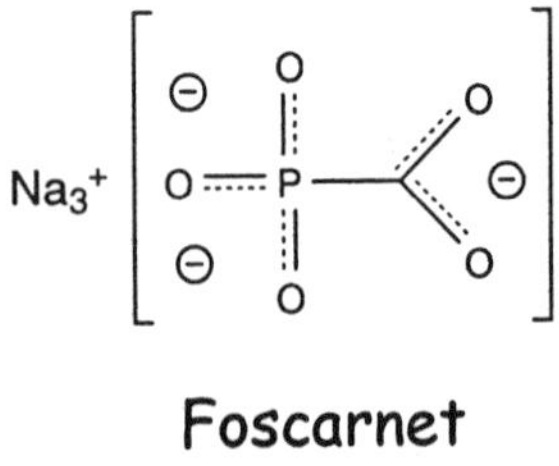

Foscarnet

Fig. 5.1.3

TRIFLURIDINE

Trifluridine is a pyrimidine analog that competitively inhibits DNA polymerase, but does not require activation by viral thymidine kinase. Thus, it is active against viruses that are resistant due to thymidine kinase deficiency. Poor selectivity for virally infected cells limits its application to the topical treatment of corneal infections with HSV.

5.1.3 Foscarnet

Identity (**Fig. 5.1.3**)

An organic analog of pyrophosphate.

Mechanism

Selectively binds to viral DNA polymerase and prevents the cleavage of pyrophosphate from nucleoside triphosphates during DNA polymerization.

Activity

CMV, acyclovir-resistant forms of HSV and VZV.

Administration, Metabolism, and Elimination

Not absorbed by the gastrointestinal tract. Eliminated by the kidneys, but kinetics complicated due to deposition in bone.

Adverse Effects

Nephrotoxicity, hypocalcemia, and hypomagnesemia from chelation of Ca^{2+} and $Mg,^{2+}$ and CNS disturbances.

Drug Interactions

Concomitant pentamidine therapy increases risk of hypocalcemia.

Resistance

Point mutations in viral DNA polymerase have caused resistance.

5.2 Antiinfluenzavirus Agents

Influenza viruses have eight segments of negative-sense single-stranded RNA in their genomes. The nucleocapsid encasing the genome contains an ion channel protein known as M2 that mediates uncoating of the genome when the virus is exposed to low pH. The nucleocapsid is surrounded by a lipid bilayer envelope. Large numbers of two different "spike" proteins are anchored in the envelope and protrude from its surface. The hemagglutinin mediates initial attachment of the virus to host cells (**Fig. 5.2**). Following attachment, endocytosis, and acidification, the hemagglutinin undergoes a structural rearrangement that releases the nucleocapsid from its envelope. The neuraminidase helps prevent viral aggregation, facilitates release from host cells, and may have a role as a virulence factor. Sequence variations and mutations in the hemagglutinin and neuraminidase spike proteins are responsible for antigenic "shift" and "drift" that enables influenza to circumvent immunity and cause epidemic disease.

5.2.1 Amantadine, Rimantadine

Identity (**Fig. 5.2.1**)

Closely related polyhedrally-shaped compounds.

Mechanism

Both drugs possess a dual mechanism of action. At an early step in viral replication, they block the function of the M2 ion channel protein. At a later stage, they interfere with hemagglutinin processing.

Activity

Influenza A only. Rimantadine is 10-fold more active than amantadine. Amantadine also has antiparkinsonism activity.

Administration, Metabolism, and Elimination

Both drugs are well absorbed and achieve high concentrations in epithelial secretions. Amantadine is eliminated unchanged in the urine, whereas rimantadine is extensively metabolized.

Adverse Effects

Minor CNS and gastrointestinal disturbances.

Influenza Virus Replication cycle

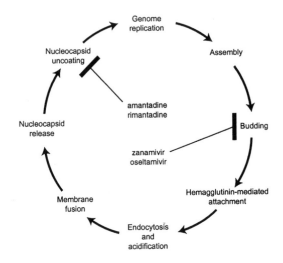

The virus binds to target cell membranes via hemagglutinins anchored in its membrane. The bound virus is then internalized by endocytosis. Within the endocytotic vesicle, lowered pH triggers a hemagglutinin-mediated membrane fusion event that releases the viral nucleocapsid into the cytosol. Disassembly of the nucleocapsid or "uncoating" of the genome is required prior to genome replication. Replicated virions are assembled in the cytoplasm and acquire their lipid envelopes upon budding through on the host cell membrane. The viral envelopes contain two main protein species: the hemagglutinin by which the virus attaches to target cells, and initiates fusion of its envelope with the endosomal membrane, and neuraminidase - an enzyme believed to prevent viral aggregation and assist with release of the virus from host cells.

Amantadine and rimantadine interfere with the function of M2, an ion channel protein involved in nucleocapsid uncoating, and may also interfere with other steps in the replication cycle. Oseltamivir and zanamivir inhibit neuraminidase activity.

Fig. 5.2

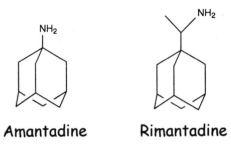

Amantadine   Rimantadine

Fig. 5.2.1

Drug Interactions.

No consistent interactions of major clinical importance.

Resistance

Mutations in the M2 protein confer resistance.

5.2.2 Oseltamivir, Zanamivir

Identity

Oseltamivir is an orally administered prodrug that must be activated by ester hydrolysis; zanamivir is inhaled in its active form. (**Fig. 5.2.2**).

Mechanism

Both drugs inhibits the neuraminidase of influenza; this interferes with viral aggregation and release from host cells.

Activity

Influenza A, possibly influenza B.

Administration, Metabolism, and Elimination

Oseltamivir is well absorbed, rapidly activated, and eliminated by the kidneys. Less than 20% of zanamivir reaches the systemic circulation after inhalation.

Adverse Effects

No major adverse effects known.

Drug Interactions

No consistent interactions of major clinical importance.

Neuraminidase Inhibitors

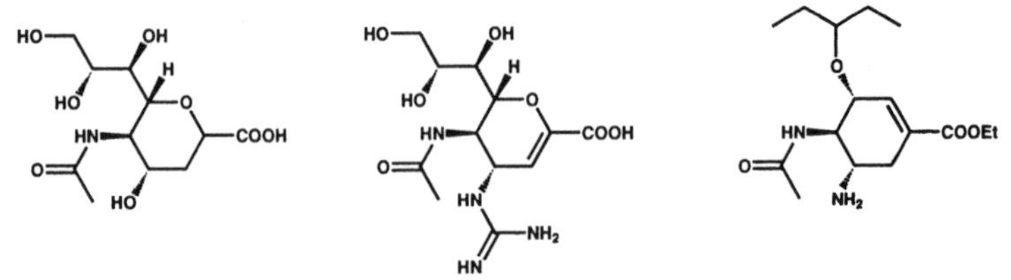

N-Acetylneuraminic acid   Zanamivir   Oseltamivir

Neuraminidase inhibitors exhibit structural similarity to N-acetylneuraminic acid, a component of many proteins in the viral and host cell membranes. Zanamivir is an active drug whereas oseltamivir is the ethyl ester of an active drug. The active drug is produced by esterases in the plasma and cells of the gut upon the absorption of oseltamivir.

Fig. 5.2.2

Resistance

Resistance due to altered viral neuraminidase has been observed.

5.3 Anti-HIV Agents (Table 5.3, Fig. 5.3)

HIV virions each have two copies of a single-stranded RNA genome, a reverse transcriptase, and an aspartic protease. Early in the viral replication cycle, reverse transciptase converts the RNA into double-stranded DNA, which is then integrated (via integrase) into the host cell DNA. The reverse transcriptase of HIV has poor fidelity, leading to frequent transcription errors, and a high degree of sequence variation among the viral genome copies that are produced. The protease catalyzes a critical step late in the viral replication cycle involving maturation of the assembled virus.

5.3.1 Reverse Transcriptase Inhibitors

Identity

Reverse transcriptase inhibitors (RTIs) are divided into two groups depending on whether or not they contain a nucleoside. Nucleoside

Table 5.3
Anti-HIV Agents

Subclass[a]	Generic name	Abbreviation	Chief toxicity
Nucleoside RTIs—pyrimidine analogs	Zidovudine	AZT	Bone marrow suppression, central nervous system disturbances, nausea
	Stavudine	d4T	Peripheral neuropathy
	Zalcitabine	ddC	Peripheral neuropathy
	lamivudine	3TC	Well tolerated
Nucleoside RTIs—purine analogs	Didanosine	ddI	Peripheral neuropathy, pancreatitis
	Abacavir	ABV	Hypersensitivity, potentially fatal
Non-nucleoside RTIs (NNRTIs)	Nevirapine	NVP	Skin rash, hepatitis
	Delavirdine	DLV	Skin rash
	Efavirenz	EFV	Central nervous system disturbances
Protease inhibitors	Saquinavir	SQV	Gastrointestinal disturbance
	Ritonavir	RTV	Gastrointestinal disturbance
	Indinavir	IDV	Crystalluria
	Nelfinavir	NFV	Gastrointestinal disturbance
	Amprenavir	APV	Gastrointestinal disturbance
	Lopinavir	LPV	Gastrointestinal disturbance

[a]RTIs—reverse transcriptase inhibitors

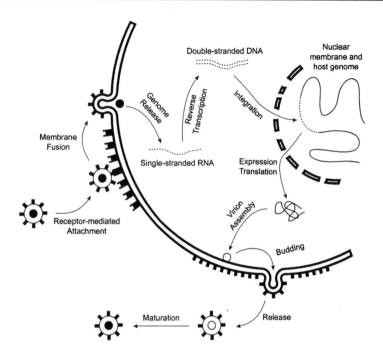

Replication cycle for HIV. There are two sites of pharmacological attack on this cycle. Reverse transcriptase inhibitors block the conversion of single stranded RNA into double-stranded DNA. These drugs prevent viruses from integrating into the host genome and completing the infection process, but they do not inhibit viral replication once integration has occurred. Protease inhibitors block a proteolytic event that is essential for capsid maturation. These drugs prevent newly-assembled virus from becoming infectious, but they do not inhibit infection by viruses that have already matured. Drugs that prevent viral attachment and that prevent integration of the viral genome are in development.

Fig. 5.3

reverse transcriptase inhibitors (NRTIs, **Fig. 5.3.1.1**) bind to the target enzyme by mimicking naturally occurring nucleosides. Non-nucleoside reverse transcriptase inhibitors (NNRTIs, **Fig. 5.3.1.2**) bind to the target enzyme in a slightly different manner. For this reason, there is little cross-resistance between these two groups among viruses, whereas cross-resistance is common within these groups.

Mechanism

NRTIs (but not NNRTIs) must be phosphorylated by host cell enzymes before becoming active. RTIs inhibit HIV reverse transcriptase, but they are also substrates. When incorporated into DNA they terminate synthesis because they lack 3'-OH groups. Reverse transcription is an early event in the replication cycle, so these agents have no effect on a cell in later stages of viral infection.

Hydroxyurea is often co-administered with the purine analogs (ddI or abacavir) to inhibit ribonucleotide reductase. This decreases the intracellular pool of adenine nucleotides, and thereby potentiates the effect of the purine analogs.

Activity

HIV-1 and HIV-2. Lamivudine also has activity against hepatitis B.

Administration, Metabolism, and Elimination

Wide variation in all parameters across this class of drugs.

Adverse Effects

The tendency to produce specific side effects varies considerably among the reverse transcriptase inhibitors, but as a class they are associated with bone marrow depression, peripheral neuropathies, and pancreatitis. Lamivudine tends to cause fewer adverse effects than other NRTIs, probably because, in addition to differing chemically from cytidine, it is also a stereoisomer **(Fig. 5.3.1.1)**.

Drug Interactions

None of major clinical significance.

Resistance

Single mutations in reverse transcriptase confer phenotypic resistance to some RTIs, while multiple mutations are required to produce phenotypic resistance to others. Cross resistance among agents in

Nucleoside Reverse Transcriptase Inhibitors (NRTIs)

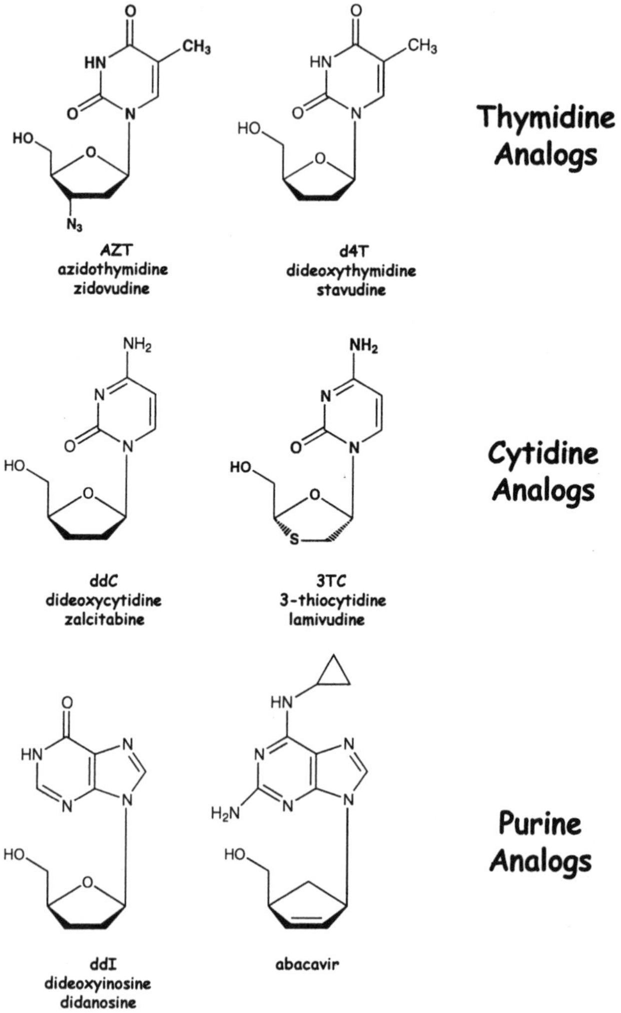

Thymidine Analogs

AZT
azidothymidine
zidovudine

d4T
dideoxythymidine
stavudine

Cytidine Analogs

ddC
dideoxycytidine
zalcitabine

3TC
3-thiocytidine
lamivudine

Purine Analogs

ddI
dideoxyinosine
didanosine

abacavir

Fig. 5.3.1.1

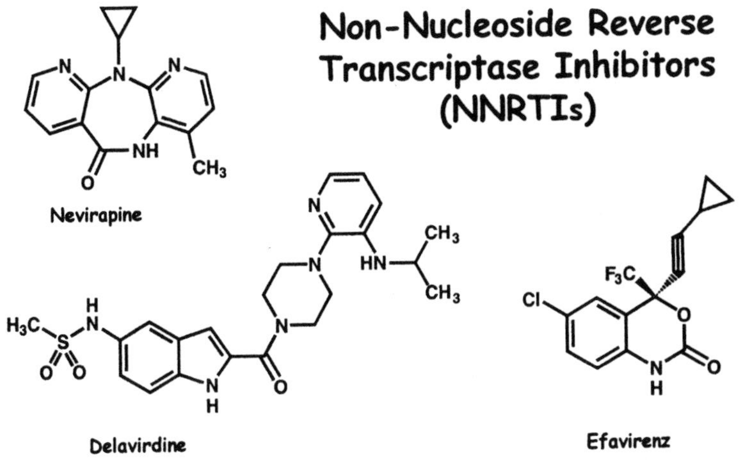

Fig. 5.3.1.2

this class is common. Mutations can also accumulate, conferring phenotypic resistance to all RTIs.

5.3.2 Protease Inhibitors

Identity

There are currently six drugs in this class approved for clinical use. Their design and development followed determination of a crystal structure for their common target, the aspartic protease of HIV (**Fig. 5.3.2**).

Mechanism (**Fig. 5.3.2**)

HIV protease inhibitors prevent the proteolytic cleavage of Gag–Pol protein by the aspartic protease that is required for maturation of the fully assembled viruses. Normally, the aspartic protease performs its proteolytic cleavages as the virus is budding from the cell membrane, or shortly thereafter (**Fig. 5.3**). Without these cleavages, the newly produced virus is not infectious.

Activity

HIV protease inhibitors are active against both HIV-1 and HIV-2 viruses. They are inactive against the human aspartic proteases renin

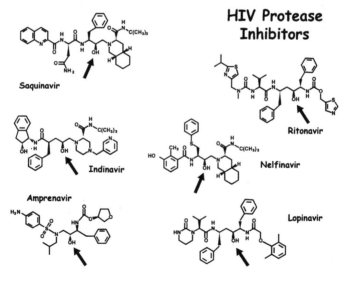

The active site of HIV protease is formed by two aspartic acid side chains at the interface of two identical monomeric subunits. These side chains create an acidic attack on a carbonyl group in the target polypeptide chain (above, left). Protease inhibitors work by filling the active site with an acid-resistant -OH group (above, right). Protease inhibitors have varied structures, but each has in common a single acid-resistant -OH group (below, arrows). Other portions of the inhibitor position this -OH group in the active site.

Fig. 5.3.2

and pepsin. All current recommendations specify that they be used in conjunction with inhibitors of HIV reverse transcriptase to avoid the emergence of resistance.

Administration, Metabolism, and Elimination

Only oral formulations are available. Oral bioavailability varies widely among individuals, and in relationship to meals. All of these drugs are metabolized by CYP_{450} enzymes in the liver. They have differing abilities to induce and/or inhibit these enzymes, and this has major effects on their plasma levels.

Adverse Effects

Various forms of gastrointestinal disturbance, elevated liver enzymes, and a peculiar redistribution of body fat are common. Crystalluria is a serious problem that is peculiar to indinavir, owing to its relatively low level of protein binding (60–65%).

Drug Interactions

The tendency of ritonavir to increase the plasma levels of saquinavir by several-fold makes these two drugs a popular combination because adequate saquinavir levels are otherwise difficult to achieve. Lopinavir is only available in combination with ritonavir for the same reason.

Resistance

The use of HIV protease inhibitors as single agents against HIV leads to the development of high level drug resistance. Each drug tends to induce characteristic single-site mutations in the protease that confer low level resistance to that drug. High-level resistance to some agents requires two mutations, and there is overlap among the secondary mutations that cause resistance to the various drugs.

5.4 Miscellaneous Agents

5.4.1 Interferons

Identity

Interferons comprise a family of potent immunoregulatory cytokines that are synthesized in response to viral infection and cause biochemical changes that inhibit viral propagation. Interferons used clinically are recombinant proteins.

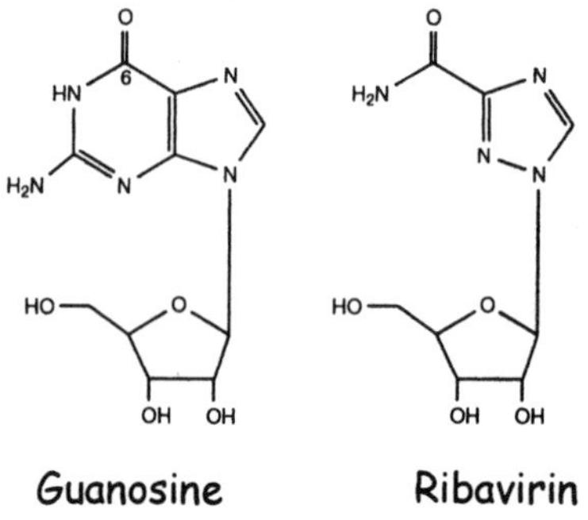

Guanosine   Ribavirin

Fig. 5.4.2

Mechanism

Multiple mechanisms of action with varying antiviral potency.

Activity

Active against most pathological viruses, although susceptibility varies. Also used against various malignancies.

Administration, Metabolism, and Elimination

Must be parenterally administered (subcutaneously, intramuscularly, intralesional). Distribution and elimination are complex.

Adverse Effects

Influenza-like syndrome typically follows administration, including fever, headache, myalgias, and gastrointestinal disturbances.
Bone marrow suppression.

Drug Interactions

Numerous interactions due to the diverse metabolic effects of interferons.

Resistance

Poorly understood.

5.4.2 Ribavirin

Identity

A modified purine nucleoside (**Fig. 5.4.2**).

Mechanism

Ribavirin must be activated by a host cell enzyme (adenosine kinase). It appears to have multiple sites of action leading to the inhibition of viral RNA synthesis.

Activity

Active against a wide variety of DNA and RNA viruses. Chief use is for the treatment of respiratory syncytial virus (RSV) in children, but it is increasingly used against hepatitis C. Activity against influenza, Lassa fever, and hantavirus infections has been reported.

Administration, Metabolism, and Elimination

Administered as an aerosol when used against RSV. Administered orally for the treatment of hepatitis C and other viral infections. Complex route of elimination.

Adverse Effects

Potentially teratogenic and oncogenic—a theoretical risk for health care providers administering aerosolized medication.

Drug Interactions

No specific interactions known.

Resistance

None known.

6 Immunomodulators and Immunizing Agents

See **Table 6.**

6.1 Immunomodulators

6.1.1 Colony-Stimulating Factors

Colony-stimulating factors are naturally occurring glycoprotein cytokines that selectively stimulate the production of various cell lines in the bone marrow. The name is derived from the clusters or "colonies" of cells that differentiate together in the marrow.

GRANULOCYTE COLONY STIMULATING FACTOR (G-CSF, FILGRASTIM)

Daily subcutaneous treatment of G-CSF specifically increases neutrophil production over 5–7 d, although a brief decline in counts is often seen at the time treatment is initiated. The mechanism of increase appears to be a combination of increased production and shortened maturation time. G-CSF is used chiefly for accelerating the recovery of neutrophil counts after chemotherapy and bone marrow transplantation, and the benefits of therapy have been clearly demonstrated in controlled studies. G-CSF is also used to raise neutrophil counts during therapy with zidovudine, ganciclovir, and other medications associated with neutropenia. G-CSF is associated with mild bone pain in a minority of patients, but is otherwise well tolerated.

From: *Essentials of Antimicrobial Pharmacology*
By: P. H. Axelsen © Humana Press, Inc., Totowa, NJ

Table 6

Currently Marketed Immunomodulators and Vaccines

Generic name	O	IV	IM	SQ	T	Trade names
Adenovirus vaccine	X					
Antirabies serum			X			
BCG vaccine					X	
Cholera vaccine			X	X		
Diphtheria and tetanus toxoid			X	X		
Diphtheria antitoxin			X			Tetramune
Diphtheria toxoid			X			Prohibit, Infanrix
Diphtheria toxoid adsorbed			X			Tripedia
Haemophilus B conjugate vaccine			X			Comvax
Haemophilus B polysaccharide			X			Prohibit, Tetramune, Acthib, Pedvaxhib
Hepatitis B immune globulin			X			Bayhep, Hepatitis, Hep-B-Gammagee
Hepatitis B surface antigen			X			Rdna, Recombivax, Comvax, Engerix, H-B-Vax
Hepatitis B virus vaccine			X			Engerix
Immune globulin human		X	X			Respigam, Gamimune, Venoglobulin, Cytogam, Baygam, Sandoglobulin, Gammar
Influenza virus vaccine			X			Fluzone, Fluvirin, Fluogen
Interferon Alfa-2a			X			Roferon
Interferon Alfa-2b			X	X		Rebetron, Intron
Interferon Alfa-N3					X	Alferon
Interferon Alfacon-1				X		Infergen
Japanese encephalitis virus					X	Je-Vax
Lyme disease			X			Lymerix
Measles–mumps–rubella virus				X		M-M-R, M-R-Vax

Immunobiologic	O	IM	SQ	IV	T	Trade name(s)
Meningococcal polysaccharide			X			Menomune, Meningovax-Ac
Mumps virus vaccine live			X			Mumpsvax, M-M-R, Biavax
Neisseria meningitidis		X				Comvax, Pedvaxhib
Pertussis vaccine		X				Diphtheria
Pneumococcal polysaccharide		X	X			Pnu-Imune, Pneumovax
Poliomyelitis Vaccine		X	X			
Rabies immune globulin		X				Imogam, Bayrab
Rabies vaccine		X			X	Imovax
Rabies vaccine adsorbed		X				Biorab
Rubella and mumps virus vaccine			X			Biavax
Tetanus antitoxin		X	X			
Tetanus immune globulin		X	X			
Tetanus toxoid		X	X			Baytet
Typhoid vaccine	X					Infanrix, Acthib
Typhoid vi polysaccharide vaccine		X	X			Vivotif
Varicella virus vaccine live		X	X			Typhim
Varicella-zoster immune globulin		X	X			Varivax
Botulism antitoxin		X	X			Iveegam
Cytomegalovirus immune globulin		X	X	X		
Tetanus immune globulin		X			X	Cytogam

O, oral; IV, intravenous; IM, intramuscular; SQ, subcutaneous; T, topical, including preparations applied to skin, eyes, and ears.

GRANULOCYTE-MACROPHAGE COLONY STIMULATING FACTOR (GM-CSF, SARGRAMOSTIM)

Daily intravenous infusion of GM-CSF for 21 d after bone marrow transplantation specifically accelerates the recovery of neutrophil, monocyte, and eosinophil counts. The mechanism of increase appears to be a combination of increased production and prolonged circulation time. GM-CSF is used chiefly for accelerating the recovery of blood counts after bone marrow transplantation, and the benefits of therapy are clear in cases of autologous bone marrow transplants, but not in allogeneic transplants. There are theoretical concerns that GM-CSF may provoke graft-vs-host disease in allogeneic transplants, and that it may stimulate viral replication in monocytes of HIV-infected persons. GM-CSF is associated with more common and more severe toxicity than G-CSF.

OTHER

Three-times-per-week subcutaneous or intravenous treatment with erythropoietin is helpful in the treatment of anemia caused by therapy with zidovudine or other drugs. Macrophage colony-stimulating factor and multicolony stimulating factor or interleukin-3 are in development.

6.1.2 Interferons

Interferons are a heterogeneous group of cytokines that are produced by leukocytes and fibroblasts in response to viral infections, certain bacterial infections, and bacterial toxins. They act synergistically with interleukins to stimulate the immune response, but they also cause multiple adverse effects including flu-like symptoms, gastrointestinal, and CNS disturbances.

ALPHA INTERFERONS

Alfa-2a and alfa-2b are homogeneous recombinant preparations. Alfa-n1 and alfa-n3 are purified mixtures. The alpha interferons are used in the treatment of chronic non-A/B/C hepatitis, hepatitis C, diverse malignancies, and myeloproliferative disorders. Alfa-2b is used to treat chronic hepatitis B infections.

BETA INTERFERONS

Beta Interferons beta-1a and beta-1b are used for multiple sclerosis.

Gamma Interferons reduce the incidence of infection in patients with chronic granulomatous disease (CGD). They are also believed to be of benefit in the treatment of visceral leishmaniasis, leprosy, and disseminated mycobacterium–avium complex.

6.1.3 Interleukins

Interleukin-2 appears to benefit patients with disseminated cutaneous leishmaniasis, leprosy, and various malignancies.

6.2 Immunization

A recommendation to immunize implies that the risk of an adverse reaction is judged to be significantly less than the risk of the disease being vaccinated against. Nevertheless, immunizations are associated with many adverse effects ranging from local reactions (pain, swelling) and moderate systemic illness (fever, myalgias), to severe life-threatening reactions (anaphylaxis, Guillain-Barré syndrome). Persons with bleeding disorders, of course, are at risk for hematoma formation at the site of innoculation. Life-threatening or even severe reactions are rare, and aside from known hypersensitivity to a particular vaccine component, it has not been possible to identify subpopulations at risk.

6.2.1 Active

Active immunization is aimed at the prevention of infectious disease by inducing immunity. Owing to the delay in response, active immunization is not an option for the treatment of active disease.

LIVE ATTENUATED VACCINES

Viruses typically infect only specific cell types, and often are able to infect these cells in a limited number of host species. By taking a human-derived virus and passaging it in animals or nonhuman cell lines that permit hindered propagation, mutations can accumulate that adapt the virus to these conditions, while at the same time reducing the virulence of the virus for its original human target. Viruses that have been altered in this way are known as "attenuated" strains, and they are used when killed forms of the original virus are not sufficiently immunogenic to provide effective or long-lasting immunity. The same basic principle was applied by Jenner, who used cowpox virus to immunize humans against smallpox.

Vaccination with live organisms may be associated with significant risks for immunocompromised patients because the course of infection with an attenuated strain may not be as benign as in immunocompetent patients. In general, killed/inactivated vaccines are preferred in these patients when available. Live vaccines generally require careful storage and handling to preserve efficacy.

Adenovirus

Available against a limited number of strains for military use.

Bacillus Calmette-Guérin

Bacillus Calmette-Guérin is a strain of *Mycobacterium bovis* that results in a significant reduction in the incidence of *Mycobacterium tuberculosis* when used to immunize a population at high risk. Because it is not completely protective, there are only rare indications for its use in countries where the incidence of *M. tuberculosis* is relatively low. A disadvantage to its use in such countries is that it causes a false-positive purified protein derivative (PPD), skin test for tuberculosis and a valuable diagnostic screening test is lost.

Measles, Mumps, Rubella

Live attenuated virus vaccines are available for separate immunization against these three illnesses, but they are most often combined and administered as a series of two injections given to children. Maternal antibodies in children less than 6 mo of age, immune globulin, and transfusions can render the vaccine ineffective. Women of childbearing age who are not immune to rubella should be vaccinated and avoid pregnancy for at least 3 mo to minimize the risk of fetal abnormalities due to rubella infection.

Recipients of a killed measles vaccine between 1963 and 1967 are susceptible to a severe atypical form of measles. These patients should be immunized with a current live-virus preparation.

Polio

Oral polio vaccine (OPV) offers easily administered, highly effective, and low-cost protection against all three serotypes of poliovirus. In addition, vaccine-strain viruses are shed by recipients through the gastrointestinal tract, thereby potentially exposing and immunizing others. However, OPV administration is not suitable for patients with impaired immunity. Most cases of poliomyelitis in the United States are now associated with OPV administration, a finding on which the current policy of using only inactivated polio vaccine is based (see later).

Smallpox

Since smallpox has been eradicated, this vaccine no longer has indications because risk of the vaccine outweighs the risk of disease.

Oral Typhoid

The vaccine consists of live bacteria in enteric coated capsules that protect the bacteria from destruction in the stomach. The capsules must be carefully stored to preserve efficacy, and patients must not be taking antibiotics concomitantly. Overall efficacy is estimated to be 50–80%.

Yellow Fever

Vaccination is required for travel to countries where yellow fever is endemic and is highly recommended because of minimal side effects, high efficacy, and the severity of disease.

Varicella

Effective at preventing chickenpox in children, and advisable for older patients without a history of chickenpox for whom primary infection can be severe. The incidence of subsequent shingles is unknown, but appears to be low.

KILLED VACCINES

Killed vaccines tend to have more complex compositions than live vaccines, and they are more likely to induce hypersensitivity reactions or other adverse effects in recipients. In addition, they tend to contain preservatives and antibiotics with the potential to induce hypersensitivity reaction.

Cholera

Although disease is caused by an enterotoxin, efforts to create a toxin-based vaccine have been unsuccessful. The current vaccine consists of inactivated *Vibrio cholera* 01 strain, and offers only unreliable partial protection for intervals of a few months. It is ineffective against other strains prevalent in Asia. There are few indications for this vaccine.

Hepatitis A

A highly effective vaccine that may be given concurrently with intramuscular immune globulin without loss of efficacy.

Influenza

Influenza types A and B are associated with epidemic and frequently severe respiratory disease. These viruses exhibit periodic minor changes in their genetic makeup and antigenic features (antigenic drift), as well as less frequent major changes (antigenic shift). The genetic makeup of viral strains most likely to cause disease in the United States can be predicted months in advance by surveillance of viral strains found in Asia. Each year, vaccine preparations are reformulated to immunize against the strains identified by surveillance, and persons at risk must be revaccinated.

Various vaccine preparations consist of inactivated whole viruses, disrupted virus particles, or purified antigens from viral cultures. The latter two preparations are known as "split-virus" preparations, and have a lower incidence of febrile reactions.

The viruses are cultured in eggs, and hypersensitivity reactions to egg proteins are possible. Various preparations also contain preservatives (mercury, thimerosol), antibiotics (aminoglycosides, polymyxin), and sulfites to which patients may have hypersensitivity reactions.

Japanese Encephalitis

This is a mosquito-borne virus and the leading cause of encephalitis in Asia. The vaccine is recommended for travelers who plan extended stays in rural areas during transmission seasons (varies with region).

Pertussis

A new "acellular" vaccine formulation is available that has fewer adverse effects than the former killed whole-cell preparation. This vaccine is almost always administered in combination with diphtheria and tetanus vaccines.

Plague

A plague vaccine is available, but it has few indications because post-exposure prophylaxis with oral antibiotics is effective.

Pneumococcus

This vaccine consists of 23 strains of *Streptococcus penumoniae* with antigenically distinct polysaccharide capsules. It is generally given only once to each patient, although revaccination of high-risk individuals to boost immunity may be appropriate.

Polio

Inactivated polio vaccine (IPV) has seen increasing use as an attempt to reduce the incidence of poliomyelitis associated with the live-virus OPV. As world health efforts make progress toward worldwide eradication of polio virus, it is anticipated that the use of IPV will completely supplant the use of OPV.

Rabies

This vaccine is used alone for preexposure prophylaxis in persons at high risk for rabies (e.g. veterinarians, certain travelers). There are two equally effective formulations: human diploid cell vaccine (HDCV) and rabies vaccine adsorbed (RVA). This vaccine is used along with rabies immune globulin for post-exposure prophylaxis.

Typhoid (Parenteral)

Vaccination with a killed strain of *S. typhi* has an estimated efficacy between 51% and 77% after two doses. The purified polysaccharide vaccine is now preferred because of fewer side effects.

COMPONENT AND TOXOID VACCINES

These vaccines typically contain aluminum hydroxide as an adjuvant. The immunogenic material is said to be "adsorbed" to the aluminum adjuvant, and this renders it more likely to induce a strong immune reaction. The presence of aluminum makes it necessary to administer these vaccines by intramuscular injection because of adverse reactions to aluminum associated with intravenous or subcutaneous administration.

Anthrax

Anthrax vaccine is made by filtering the culture medium in which an avirulent nonencapsulated strain of *Bacillus anthracis* has been grown, and adsorbing the toxin onto aluminum hydroxide. Even with adjuvant, however, the development of effective immunity requires multiple innoculations, and the maintenance of immunity requires periodic reinoculation. For obvious reasons, testing the efficacy of the vaccine by challenging people with lethal organisms is not possible, but the vaccine appears to confer effective immunity in animals.

Diphtheria, Tetanus, Pertussis (DTP)

In all of its forms, DTP is the most widely administered of all vaccines. All three diseases, against which this vaccine is targeted, are mediated by toxins. Diphtheria is caused by a toxin elaborated by *Corynebacterium diphtheriae*. This is a ubiquitous bacterium that becomes toxigenic upon infection with a specific bacteriophage. Tetanus ("lockjaw") is caused by a toxin produced by *Clostridium tetani*, another ubiquitous soil bacterium. Pertussis ("whooping cough") is caused by a toxin produced by *Bordetella pertussis*.

The tetanus and diphtheria toxins are chemically treated to form nontoxic but immunogenic "toxoids," and are adsorbed onto aluminum hydroxide. They may be administered without the pertussis component (DT = pediatric formulation, dT = adult "booster" formation).

The pertussis component is available in two forms. DTP (or DTwP) contains an inactivated whole-cell preparation of *B. pertussis* bacteria. More recently, an acellular adsorbed form (DTaP) has become available, and is associated with fewer adverse reactions.

Hemophilus

There are six antigenically distinct polysaccharide capsules among strains of *Hemophilus influenzae*. Capsules designated type "b" are most often associated with invasive disease (e.g., meningitis) in children, although many children are immune by age 5–6 yr as a result of asymptomatic exposure.

The vaccine consists of capsular polysaccharide chemically conjugated to a protein carrier to improve immunogenicity. In some cases, the protein carrier is tetanus or diphtheria toxoid. These preparations are effective at immunizing against *H. influenzae*, but not approved for vaccination against tetanus or diptheria.

Hepatitis B

Hepatitis B virus (HBV) infection generally results in the development of antibodies to surface, core, and "e" antigens. The presence of antibodies to surface antigens is protective against infection, and early formulations of the vaccine consisted of purified surface antigen from persons with chronic hepatitis B. Current vaccines are made from recombinant surface antigen produced by yeast and adsorbed to aluminum adjuvant. Hypersensitivity reactions to yeast protein are possible.

Persons immunized with HBV vaccine will have measurable antibody titers to hepatitis B surface antigen (HBsAb), but not core or e antigens. Persons with a history of HBV infection are serologically distinct because they will also have antibodies to core and possibly e antigens.

Lyme Disease

Lyme disease vaccine is composed of a recombinant form of outer surface protein A from *B. burgdorferi* (rOsp-A). This organism undergoes a major antigenic change between the time of tick attachment on a mammalian host and subsequent transmission of the bacterium to the host. The spirochetes residing in the tick gut at the initiation of tick feeding express primarily OspA. As tick feeding begins, OspA is largely replaced by OspC so that spirochetes reaching a mammalian host after passing through the tick salivary glands express primarily OspC. Since the rOsp-A vaccine does work, it is believed that the antibodies it elicits kill Lyme disease spirochetes within the tick gut (i.e., not within the host).

Lyme disease vaccine has not been recommended for widespread use because it is not fully protective, and it causes false-positive diagnostic tests (ELISA, but not Western blot). Because the risk of disease for most people is low, it has also been criticized on cost-benefit grounds.

Meningococcus

There are at least eight serologically distinct polysaccharide capsules among pathological strains of *Neisseria meningitidis*. The vaccine consists of purified capsular antigens from strains A, C, Y, and W-135. Strain B is a common cause of meningitis in the United States, and is not included in the vaccine.

Typhoid (Parenteral)

A purified polysaccharide extracted from capsules of a strain of *S. typhi* is available with an efficacy estimated to be 55–74% after a single dose and 90% after two doses. This vaccine has fewer side effects and fewer doses required than the killed bacteria vaccine.

6.2.2 Passive

Passive immunization is used in three circumstances: when immediate immunity is needed, when active immunization is not available, or when the patient is not capable of mounting an immune response.

NONSPECIFIC

Ig for hepatitis A

A preparation for intramuscular use made from purified human immunoglobulin fractions with relatively high titers of antibody to hepatitis A. It is effective for short-term pre- and post-exposure prophylaxis against hepatitis A. It does not reduce the efficacy of killed hepatitis A vaccine, and both may be given concurrently.

Intravenous Ig

A preparation for intravenous use made from purified human immunoglobulin fractions for the treatment of immunoglobulin deficiency, immune thrombocytopenic purpura, and Kawasaki disease. May be of some use in postexposure prophylaxis against infections in immunoglobulin-deficient patients, but should not to be used for prophylaxis against hepatitis A.

SPECIFIC

CMV

Prepared from human plasma with high titers of cytomegalovirus antibody for post-exposure prophylaxis.

Hepatitis B

Prepared from human plasma with high titers of hepatitis B surface antibody for post-exposure prophylaxis.

Rabies

A hyperimmune immunoglobulin fraction prepared from actively immunized animals. Used for post-exposure prophylaxis against rabies. In cases of rabies exposure via skin wound, the wound should be cleansed with soapy water (highly effective at inactivating the virus) and infiltrated with half of the recommended dose of rabies immune globulin (the other half is administered intramuscularly).

Rh factor

For use in Rh-negative women who have delivered Rh-positive babies to avoid sensitization of the mother to Rh antigen at the time of delivery.

Tetanus

Available for post-exposure prophylaxis and treatment.

Vaccinia

Intended for use in treating complications of smallpox vaccination. No current indications.

Varicella-Zoster

Prepared from human plasma with high titers of antibody to varicella-zoster virus for post-exposure prophylaxis.

Index

Bacampicillin, 14
Baciim, 50
Bacillus anthracis, 117
Bacillus Calmette-Guérin, 114
Bacitracin, 33, 50, 52, 53
Bacter-Aid, 29
Bacteriocidal, 2, 7
Bacteriostatic, 2
Bactocill, 14
Bactramycin, 37
Bactrim, 29
Bactroban, 50
Balantidium coli, 76
Baygam, 110
Bayhep, 110
Bayrab, 111
Baytet, 111
BCG vaccine, 110
Beepen, 14
Benzathine penicillin, 14
Benznidazole, 83
Benzodiazepines, 72
β-lactamase, 20, 21, 22, 24, 59
β-lactamase inhibitor, 22
β-lactams, 11, 16, 17, 18, 19, 20,
    21, 22, 24, 26, 57, 59, 60
Bethaprim, 29
Biavax, 111
Biaxin, 36
Bicillin, 14
Bile, 5, 39, 44
Biliary tract, 4
Biltricide, 74
Bioavailability, 2, 4, 17, 38, 42, 49,
    83, 105
Biocef, 14
Biorab, 111
Bio-Tab, 36
Blastocystis, 76

Blastomycosis, 70
Bleeding, 22
Bleph-10, 29
Blephamide, 29
Blood-brain barrier, 4, 21
Bloodstream infections, 2, 4
Bone marrow depression, 42, 92,
    101
Bordetella pertussis, 118
Borrelia, 38
Borrelia burgdorferi, 119
Botulism antitoxin, 111
Bradycardia, 79
Broad-spectrum, 1, 12
Brodspec, 36
Bronchospasm, 81
Brucella, 34
Brugia malayi (filariasis), 76
Bubonic plague, 34
Budding, 96
Butoconazole, 66
C
Calcium, 39
Calcium channel blockers, 79
Candida, 57, 68, 70
Candidiasis, 60
Capastat, 54
Capreomycin, 54, 59
Capsular polysaccharide, 118
Capsules, 118
Carbamazepine, 41
Carbapenems, 15, 17, 19, 21, 24
Carbenicillin, 14
Carbenicillinase, 22
Carrier mechanisms, 3, 13, 16, 32,
    35, 38, 39, 41, 43
Cartilage, 49
Caspofungin, 72
Cavitary tuberculosis, 54, 59

Interstitial nephritis, 22
Intrathecal administration, 4, 67
Intravascular compartment, 4
Intravesicle administration, 67
Intron, 110
Investigational agents, 60
Invirase, 88
Iodoquinol, 74, 78
Ipecac, 74
IPV, 117
Isoleucine, 52
Isoniazid (INH), 54, 55, 57
Isospora belli, 76
Itraconazole, 66, 70, 71
Iveegam, 111
Ivermectin, 74, 84, 85
J
Japanese encephalitis, 110, 116
Jarish-Herxheimer reaction, 19
Je-Vax, 110
Joint spaces, 6
K
Kaletra, 88
Kanamycin, 32, 33, 58
Kantrex, 33
Keflex, 14
Keftab, 14
Keftabs, 14
Kefurox, 15
Kefzol, 14
Keratinocytes, 72
Ketek, 37
Ketoconazole, 66, 70, 71
Ketolides, 37, 41
Killed vaccines, 115
Klaron, 29
L
Lactam, 17
Lactam ring, 17

Lactobacillus, 27
Lactobionate, 36, 40
Lamisil, 66
Lamivudine, 88, 99, 101, 102
Lamprene, 54
Lariam, 74
Lassa fever, 107
Latent infection, 55, 56, 57
Legionella, 40
Leishmania, 34, 65, 76, 81, 83, 113
Leprosy, 31, 113
Levaquin, 47
Levofloxacin, 47, 48
Lincocin, 37
Lincoject, 37
Lincomycin, 37
Linezolid, 37, 38, 45
Lipid vesicles, 67
Lipopeptide antibiotic, 60
Liposomal preparations, 67
Liposomes, 67
Lipoteichoic acid synthesis, 60
Live-attenuated vaccines, 113
Loa loa (African eye worm), 76
Lockjaw, 118
Lomefloxacin, 47
Lopinavir (LPV), 88, 99, 104, 105
Loprox, 66
Lorabid, 15
Loracarbef, 15
Loram, 41
Lotrimin, 66
Lotrisone, 66
LPV, 99
Luminal protozoa, 73
Lyme disease, 19, 21, 110, 119
Lymerix, 110
Lytic enzymes, 13

Valacyclovir, 88, 89, 91
Valcyte, 88
Valganciclovir, 88, 89, 91
Valtrex, 88
Vancocin, 15
Vancoled, 15
Vancomycin, 27
Vancomycin-resistant *Enterococci*,
 16, 28, 42, 45, 46, 61
Vantin, 15
Varicella virus vaccine live, 111
Varicella-zoster immune globulin,
 111, 121
Varicella-zoster virus (VZV), 88,
 91, 115
Varivax, 111
Vasocidin, 29
Vasosulf, 29
Vectrin, 36
Veetids, 14
Vegetations, 5, 6
Velosef, 14
Venoglobulin, 110
Verapamil, 79
Vermox, 74
Vestibular nerve, 35
Vestibular toxicity, 58
Veterinarians, 117
Vibramycin, 36
Vibra-Tabs, 36
Vibrio cholera, 115
Vidarabine, 88
Videx, 88
Viomycin, 59
Vira-A, 88
Viracept, 88
Viral envelope, 95

Viramune, 88
Virazole, 88
Virginiamycin, 45, 47
Viroptic, 88
Visceral larva migrans, 83
Vistide, 88
Vitamin B6, 56
Vivotif, 111
von Willebrand's disease, 26
VZV, 88, 94
W
Warfarin, 32, 41, 43
Whipworms, 83
Whole-cell vaccine, 116
Whooping cough, 118
Wuchereria bancrofti (filariasis),
 76
Wycillin, 14
X
Xanthomonas, 21, 49
Y
Yellow fever, 115
Yodoxin, 74
Z
Zagam, 47
Zalcitabine, 88, 99, 102
Zanamivir, 88, 96, 97, 98
Zefazone, 15
Zerit, 88
Ziagen, 88
Zidovudine, 88, 99, 102, 109, 112
Zinacef, 15
Zithromax, 36
Zone of inhibition, 7, 8, 9
Zosyn, 14, 24
Zovirax, 88
Zyvox, 37

'I'... ... ... er you, sir,' Faye blurted as soon as the door had closed.

'I made it obvious when you were last here that I like being bothered by you, Miss Shawcross.' Slowly he straightened ... ...rned to face her. 'In fact, I'm hoping you've saved me ... ...y to Mulberry House to speak to you. If you're back ... ...e you feel the same way about me, I can suggest ... ...e might do about it.'

T... ...ony in his voice couldn't quite disguise the fact that h... ...nt every word. And heaven only knew she *did* crave ha... ...his strong arms about her again. She knew if he b... ...d her mouth with his own, as he had before, his fiery pa... ...n would eradicate every worry from her head as easily as ...ight dissolved snow.

'I ...ice from your silence that you're in two minds on it. P... ...s I should help you decide.' He plunged his hands in ...s pockets and pinned her down with a dangerously cl... ...nging stare.

F... ...ut down her untasted tea in a rattle of crockery. 'I bid y... ...be serious, sir, if you will.'

'I ...ever been more serious in my life,' he returned.

H... ...vid, unsmiling eyes tangled with hers before travelling o... ...er body in a way that caused iced heat to streak t... ...h her veins.

'... ...neither was *I* more serious than when I told you I will s... ...be married.' Slashes of bright colour accented Faye's c... ...bones. 'You shouldn't have kissed me, Mr Kavanagh, a... ...shouldn't have…'

...ole to explain herself, she snatched up her hat and ...es from the sofa.

...shouldn't have betrayed your fiancé by liking it?' he ...sted. 'Perhaps your feelings for Mr Collins aren't as st...ng as you thought they were.'

Author Note

In my new Regency romance, *Rescued by the Forbidden Rake*, the heroine is known to be a *good* young woman. Everybody says so. Faye Shawcross has cared for her younger half-siblings since their feckless widowed mother abandoned them to chase after her lover. She's also been a constant fiancée to her seafaring future husband.

But sometimes the temptation to stray from the path of righteousness is too strong to resist. Especially when it becomes obvious that duty and selflessness are not appreciated by those benefiting from them. Faye might be sweet-natured, but she is nobody's doormat!

For years Faye has been content to settle for the quiet life of a country lady, surrounded by pastoral beauty and good friends. When Viscount Ryan Kavanagh turns up in the neighbourhood gossip immediately starts about this handsome Irishman's licentious ways.

The things that Faye hears about Valeside Manor's new squire can't *possibly* be true…can they? He seems to be the perfect neighbour, helping her out of one tricky situation after another when her younger sister falls in love with a gypsy lad. But has Ryan Kavanagh an ulterior motive where she's concerned, that proves his devilishness isn't simply a rumour? And who is he *really*, anyway?

Faye wants to believe her rescuer sincere, but how can she trust him when he is reluctant to tell her about himself? Should she jeopardise everything she holds dear and take a chance on a future with the wicked Irishman?

I hope you enjoy reading about how Faye and Ryan battle their way through lies and deceit to discover peace and happiness for themselves and their families.